Community Oral Health Practice

for the Dental Hygienist

Community Oral Health Practice

for the Dental Hygienist

Kathy Voigt Geurink, RDH, MA
Clinical Associate Professor
Department of Dental Hygiene
School of Allied Health Sciences
University of Texas Health Science Center
  at San Antonio
San Antonio, Texas

W.B. SAUNDERS COMPANY
An Imprint of Elsevier Science
Philadelphia London New York St. Louis Sydney Toronto

W.B. SAUNDERS COMPANY
An Imprint of Elsevier Science

The Curtis Center
Independence Square West
Philadelphia, Pennsylvania 19106

Library of Congress Cataloging-in-Publication Data

Geurink, Kathy Voigt.
  Community oral health practice for the dental hygienist/Kathy Voigt Geurink.—1st ed.,

  p. cm.

  ISBN 0–7216–9044–0

  1. Dental public health. 2. Community dental services. 3. Dental hygienists. I. Title.

RK52 .G48 2002

362.1'976—dc21   2001020298

Editor-in-Chief: Andrew Allen
Acquisitions Editor: Shirley Kuhn
Developmental Editor: Helaine Tobin
Project Manager: Tina Rebane
Manuscript Editor: Carol J. Robins
Illustration Specialist: John Needles
Book Designer: Marie Gardocky Clifton

COMMUNITY ORAL HEALTH PRACTICE FOR THE DENTAL HYGIENIST   ISBN 0–7216–9044–0

Copyright © 2002 by W.B. Saunders Company

Printed in the United States of America

Last digit is the print number: 9   8   7   6   5   4   3   2

This text is dedicated to dental health professionals who have participated in community efforts to improve the oral health of all citizens. Oral health, as an integral component of the overall health and well-being of individuals, must be an entity available and attainable by all populations. Throughout my many years of working in the field of community oral health, I have observed the dedication and commitment of dental health professionals working toward this goal. They need to be commended and thanked and told to keep up their efforts. Many worthwhile programs and services have been provided, but there is still much to be done.

Contributors

Linda Altenhoff, DDS
Dental Director
Division of Oral Health, Texas Department of Health
Public Health Region 8
Headquarters: Austin, Texas
   Oral Health Programs in the Community

Diane Brunson, RDH, MPH
Director, Oral Health
Colorado Department of Public Health and Environment
Clinical Assistant Professor
University of Colorado, School of Dentistry
Denver, Colorado
   Social Responsibility

Kathy Voigt Geurink, RDH, MA
Clinical Associate Professor
Department of Dental Hygiene
School of Allied Health Sciences
University of Texas Health Science Center at San Antonio
San Antonio, Texas
   *People's Health; Careers in Public Health for the Dental Hygienist; Oral Health
   Programs in the Community; Test-Taking Strategies and Community Cases*

Beverly Isman, RDH, MPH
Private Dental Public Health Consultant
Davis, California
   Health Promotion and Health Communication

Sherry Jenkins, RDH, BS
Public Health Dental Hygienist
Division of Oral Health, Texas Department of Health
Public Health Region 8
Headquarters: Austin, Texas
   Oral Health Programs in the Community

Sharon Logue, RDH, MPH
Assistant Professor and Local Coordinator, Dental Hygiene
Virginia Western Community College/Lord Fairfax Community College
Joint Venture Dental Hygiene Program
Middletown, Virginia
Careers in Public Health for the Dental Hygienist

Stacy Long, RDH, MS
Associate Project Manager
PPD Development
Austin, Texas
Research

Jane E.M. Steffensen, RDH, MPH, CHES, BS
Assistant Professor
Department of Community Dentistry, Dental School
University of Texas Health Science Center at San Antonio
San Antonio, Texas
Assessment in the Community; Measuring Progress in Oral Health

Chapter 2 Mini-Profiles by:

Kathleen Mangskau, RDH, MPA
North Dakota Department of Health
Bismarck, North Dakota

Ginger Melton, RDH, BS
Dental Program
Portsmouth City Health Department
Portsmouth, Virginia

Kathy Phipps, RDH, MPH, DrPH
Associate Professor, School of Dentistry
Research Associate Professor, School of Medicine
Oregon Health Sciences University
Portland, Oregon

Leonor Ramos, RDH
Health Educator/Wellness Promoter
Hospital Dentistry Dental Hygienist
Department of Defense
U.S. Air Force
Wilford Hall Medical Center
Lackland Air Force Base
San Antonio, Texas

Carol Marchisotto Reid, RDH
Rockingham County Health Department
Wentworth, North Carolina

JoAnn Wells, RDH, BS
Division of Dental Health
Virginia Department of Health
Richmond, Virginia

Reviewers

Chris French Beatty, RDH, PhD
Texas Women's University
Denton, Texas

Wanda Cloet, RDH, MS
Central Community College
Hastings, Nebraska

Nancy O. Cuttic, BSDH, MEd
Assistant Professor
Harcum College
Bryn Mawr, Pennsylvania

Alice S. Derouen, AS, BS
Director, Dental Hygiene
Department Chair, Dental Hygiene/Dental Assisting
Horry-Georgetown Technical College
Conway, South Carolina

Lynnette Engeswick, RDH, MS
Minnesota State University, Mankato
Mankato, Minnesota

Rita Jablon, CDA, LDH, RDH, BGS
Indiana University Northwest Dental Education
Gary, Indiana

Mary S. Pelletier, RDH, BS
Indiana River Community College
Fort Pierce, Florida

Janice Suzanne Raulerson, RDH, BSDH
Brevard Community College
Cocoa, Florida

Laura Strefling Saye, RDH, BS, MA (Couns.), MA (Sci. Ed.)
Kellogg Community College
Battle Creek, Michigan

Nanci G. Yokom, RDH, BS, MBA
Indiana University, South Bend
South Bend, Indiana

Preface

"Why do I need to know anything about Community Oral Health?"

This is the question many dental hygiene instructors hear from their dental hygiene students at the beginning of the Community Dental/Oral Health course. The purpose of this text is to provide students with information on community oral health that is relevant to dental hygiene. It is the intent of the author that, through reading the chapters and participating in the suggested activities, dental hygiene students will find the answer to this question and will develop an understanding of the importance of this integral component of their education and future profession. Although this text is written specifically for the dental hygiene student, it will also be a valuable resource for all dental hygienists practicing their professional responsibility of improving the oral health of their community.

Community Dental/Oral Health is a required course for dental hygiene accreditation. The Commission on Dental Hygiene Accreditation states that the curriculum in the dental hygiene schools must include content in the following general areas: general education, biomedical sciences, dental sciences, and dental hygiene science. These areas must be incorporated with sufficient depth, scope, sequence of instruction, quality, and emphasis to ensure achievement of the curriculum's competencies.

According to Accreditation Standard 2–14,

> *Dental hygiene science content must include oral health education and preventive counseling, health promotion, patient management, clinical dental hygiene, provision of services for and management of patients with special needs, **community dental/oral health,** medical and dental emergencies including basic life support, legal and ethical aspects of dental hygiene practice, infection and hazard control management, and the provision of oral health care services to patients with bloodborne infectious diseases.*

The American Association of Dental Schools (AADS), renamed the American Dental Education Association (ADEA), Section on Dental Hygiene Education Competency Development Committee, developed dental hygiene competencies to assist dental hygiene schools in meeting accreditation standards. The competency statements are meant to serve as guidelines for individual programs in defining the abilities they want their graduates to possess. The competency statements are presented in the following five domains:

- ◆ Core Competencies (C)
- ◆ Health Promotion/Disease Prevention (HP)
- ◆ Community (CM)
- ◆ Patient/Client Care (PC)
- ◆ Professional Growth and Development (PGD)

The ADEA Community Dental/Oral Health Competencies are as follows:

- ◆ **CM.1** Assess the oral health needs of the community and the quality of resources and services
- ◆ **CM.2** Provide screening, referral, and educational services that allow clients to access the resources of the health care system
- ◆ **CM.3** Provide community oral health services in a variety of settings
- ◆ **CM.4** Facilitate client access to oral health services by influencing individuals and organizations for the provision of oral health care
- ◆ **CM.5** Evaluate reimbursement mechanisms and their impact on the patient's or client's access to oral health care
- ◆ **CM.6** Evaluate the outcomes of community-based programs and plan for future activities

At the end of each chapter in this book, competencies from all domains that are relevant to the chapter content and knowledge application activities are listed. The complete document of competencies for entry into the profession of dental hygiene, approved and adopted by the AADS House of Delegates in 1999, is located in Appendix B. Therefore, the instructor and student will be able to relate the information within *Community Oral Health Practice for the Dental Hygienist* to the goal of developing competencies in the profession of dental hygiene.

Chapter 1 defines community oral health for the students through examples of public health problems and solutions. The core public health functions and essential public health services are defined. Chapter 2, on careers in public health, enables students to envision the future use of the information they are learning about in the book and in the community course; it features dental hygienists who practice within the field of community oral health. Reviewing these featured career choices will allow the students to comprehend the relevance of the content in the forthcoming chapters.

Chapter 3, on assessment, and Chapter 4, on measuring oral health, emphasize the importance of these crucial steps in planning community oral health programs. Dental hygienists involved in public health need to be knowledgeable of and proficient in utilizing the tools of assessment and measurement of oral health. *Healthy People 2010* oral health objectives are discussed as an important framework for assessment of community oral health programs. These chapters are appropriately placed within the book as a preparation for Chapter 5, on community oral health programs, which discusses planning, implementation, and evaluation phases of program development. Successful community oral health programs at local, state, and national levels are featured. Internet Web sites and updates on state oral health programs are included.

Chapter 6 covers statistics in a relevant, organized format, with application to community oral health. Criteria for reviewing dental literature are included. Chapter 7 explains theories of health promotion and identifies strategies for delivering health information to the public. The dental hygienist's social responsibility with respect to cultural competency and the dental hygienist's role in improving access to care for underserved populations are addressed in Chapter 8. A case study is provided to initiate discussion on the dental hygienist's roles, values, and beliefs.

Chapter 9 provides the student with practice in answering community oral health test questions similar to those on the Dental Hygiene National Board Exam. These community cases test the student's understanding of content in the textbook. The practice test will assist the student in successfully answering this type of question. Teachers using this textbook should anticipate improved scores on the national board examination in the area of community oral health. Students will be provided with the information they need to begin their profession with a positive attitude toward community dental health and a willingness to contribute to the oral health of all persons in their community.

A vocabulary of terms is unique to community oral health practice, and therefore a glossary is located at the end of the textbook for reference. The Appendices contain Web sites for oral health resources, dental hygiene competencies, and valuable information for forming community partnerships and performing community health assessments.

Bibliography

Commission on Dental Accreditation: Accreditation Standards for Dental Hygiene Education Programs (approved July 1998; effective January 2000). Chicago, American Dental Association.

American Association of Dental Schools (AADS): Competencies for Entry into the Profession of Dental Hygiene: AADS Section on Dental Hygiene Education (approved March 1999).

KATHY VOIGT GEURINK

Acknowledgments

Over the course of preparing this text for publication, many people have provided their support, guidance, and assistance in researching information pertinent to oral health in the community. I want to acknowledge with sincere appreciation the following persons for their contributions and support:

Jane Steffensen
(Colleague and Contributor)

Jill Nield-Gehrig
(Colleague and Friend)

Ray Dunham
(Network Analyst, University of Texas Health Science Center at San Antonio)

Keith Hicks
(Network Analyst, University of Texas Health Science Center at San Antonio)

Janna Lawrence
(Reference and Instructional Services Coordinator, Briscoe Library, University of Texas Health Science Center at San Antonio)

Faculty and Staff
(Department of Dental Hygiene, School of Allied Health Sciences University of Texas Health Science Center at San Antonio)

My family
(Parents, Peg and Jim Voigt
 Husband, Terry
 Daughters, Kelly and Kimberly)

Contents

People's Health

Kathy Voigt Geurink, RDH, MA

OBJECTIVES

Upon completion of this chapter, the student will be able to:

- Define the terms health, public health, and dental public health

- Identify public health problems within a community

- Identify public health measures or solutions

- Define dental disease as a public health problem with public health solutions

- Explain the role of the government in public health solutions

- Discuss the 10 greatest public health achievements of the 20th century

- Identify core functions of public health and the essential public health services

- Define six roles of the dental hygienist in order to determine how they relate to community oral health practice

Key Terms

Health

Public Health

Dental Public Health

Community

Fluoridation

Department of Health and
Human Services (DHHS)

Assessment

Policy Development

Assurance

Service Provider/Clinician

Health Educator/Wellness
Promoter

Consultant/Resource Person

Consumer
Advocate/Change Agent

Researcher

Administrator/Manager

Opening Statement

What Is Public Health?

- *Influenza immunizations save lives and money.*

- *Vaccine research of human immunodeficiency virus (HIV) is a top priority to end the epidemic.*

- *Community water fluoridation is listed as one of the 10 greatest public health achievements of the 20th century.*

- *Evidence links dental disease to life-threatening systemic diseases, such as heart disease, respiratory ailments, and diabetes.*

- *The Web site of the world's largest tobacco company acknowledges that smoking tobacco causes serious health risks.*

- *Improved water sanitation controls infectious diseases.*

- *The White House and the American Dental Hygienists Association (ADHA) team together to provide dental insurance to children.*

HEALTH, PUBLIC HEALTH, AND DENTAL PUBLIC HEALTH

Becoming familiar with the Opening Statement will set you on the right track to begin your journey in developing an understanding of the importance of people's health. The connection between people's health and community oral health will become apparent throughout the text. Thinking of specific examples, such as those in the Opening Statement, will enable you to envision what is meant by the topics of **health, public health,** and **dental public health.** It is also necessary to review the more formal definitions of these terms that occur in most texts on the topics. Various definitions exist for these terms; however, the following definitions should suffice for use within the scope of community oral health practice for the dental hygienist:

+ *Health* has been described by the World Health Organization (WHO) as follows: "Health comprises complete physical and social well-being and is not merely the absence of disease."[1]
+ *Public health,* as described by Winslow, is "the science and art of preventing disease, prolonging life, and promoting physical health and efficiency through organized community efforts."[2] It is concerned with lifestyle and behavior, the environment, human biology, and organizations of health programs and systems.[3] The **public** pertains to the community, state, or nation. Public health is people's health.[4]
+ *Dental public health* has been described by the American Board of Dental Health as

the science and art of preventing and controlling dental disease and promoting dental health through organized ***community*** *efforts. It is that form of dental practice which serves the community as the patient rather than the individual. It is concerned with the dental education of the public, and applied dental research, and with the administration of group dental care programs as well as prevention and control of dental diseases on a community basis.*[2]

In this text, the terms *public health* and *community health* are used synonymously, and both refer to the "effort that is organized by society to protect, promote and restore the health and quality of life of the people."[3]

▨ THE PUBLIC HEALTH PROBLEM AND THE PUBLIC HEALTH SOLUTION

Public Health Problem

Upon reading these definitions carefully, you are ready to view two concepts of importance to your comprehension of public or people's health: (1) the public health problem and (2) the public health solution. The public health problem, as perceived by the public, usually brings to mind an infectious disease such as acquired immunodeficiency syndrome (AIDS) or hepatitis. The spectrum of problems, however, is vast and more extensive than one might first realize. Examples of public health problems include:

1. Diseases caused by the pollution of the country's air and water systems.
2. Chronic diseases of the expanding population of older adults.
3. Inadequate funding for dental disease in indigent children.
4. An increase in violence among youth of today.

Studying examples of public health problems appears to be the easiest means of developing an understanding of what constitutes public health.

Public health problems, as described by Burt and Ecklund, must meet the following criteria[5]:

1. A condition or situation that is a widespread actual or potential cause of morbidity or mortality.
2. An existing perception that the condition is a public health problem on the part of the public, the government, or public health authorities.

The history of public health demonstrates that once the problem is identified and knowledge and expertise have been developed to solve the problem, the community must unify to find social and political support to proceed with the public health solutions.

Public Health Solution

Examples of solutions to public health problems that most persons are familiar with include immunizations, tobacco cessation programs, **fluoridation** of drinking water, and seat belts and air bags in cars to prevent injuries and mortality. These public health solutions are concerned with health promotion and disease prevention. They address the problems of the community at large and are effective measures that follow seven characteristics (see "Guiding Principles").

Guiding Principles

Seven Characteristics of Public Health Solutions

1. Not hazardous to life or function.
2. Effective in reducing or preventing the targeted disease or condition.
3. Easily and efficiently implemented.
4. Potency maintained for a substantial time period.
5. Attainable regardless of socioeconomic status.
6. Effective immediately upon application.
7. Inexpensive and within the means of the community.

Community water *fluoridation* has proved to be a safe, cost-effective solution for reducing dental decay in children. It is easily implemented by adding fluoride to the water supply, and it reaches all people regardless of socioeconomic status. It is effective immediately upon initiation and costs far less than the financial burden of restorative treatment. It meets all the seven characteristics to be considered an effective solution to the problem of dental decay.

▨ DENTAL DISEASE AS A PUBLIC HEALTH PROBLEM

Dental Decay

Dental disease is a universal problem that does not undergo remission if left untreated. About 99% of adults have had tooth decay by the time they reach their early 40s. Sixty percent of adults over 75 years of age have had root caries.[6] The extent and severity of dental caries warrant the need for treatment and prevention programs throughout the United States. Dental decay, if left untreated, continues to escalate and results in expensive surgical procedures. Therefore, it is important to focus on prevention of the disease.

Community water fluoridation is the perfect example of a dental public health solution to the problem of dental decay. Organized community efforts have brought fluoridated drinking water to more than 144 million people, and the results have shown a significant reduction in the amount of dental decay. Dental disease, however, still exists as a public health problem of the 21st century. More community dental health education needs to be performed with the implementation of additional dental health promotion and prevention programs.

Chapters 5 and 7 describe various programs and health promotion efforts that can be implemented and expanded upon within communities nationwide. The 2000 Surgeon General's report on oral health emphasizes the need for these programs and addresses the importance of oral health to the general health of the public.[6a] Dental disease is discussed as a dental public health problem of universal prevalence that can be alleviated, and even prevented, with future public health measures. Dental professionals, both those employed in the field of public health and those employed in private practice, must work together to educate the community and to provide the necessary programs to treat and prevent further disease.

Public Health/Private Practice

Programs to treat dental disease can be conducted on a *community* (public health) or *individual* (private practice) level. On the community level, the dental professional treats the community as a patient rather than as an individual. Figure 1–1 demonstrates the similarities of community oral health practice to private practice. The community oral health steps parallel steps conducted in the private practice. Community oral health practice extends the role of the dental hygienist in private practice to include the people of the community as a whole. The public health facility (e.g., hospital, community clinic, school, or agency), rather than the private dental office, becomes the environment in which the service of oral health care is provided. The patient's dental examination parallels the community survey as a means of assessment of the situation or problem.

Figure 1-1. Comparison chart of components in private practice and public health.

Private practice	Public health
• Patient	• Community
• Exam	• Survey
• Diagnosis	• Analysis
• Treatment planning	• Program planning
• Treatment	• Program implementation
• Fee/payment	• Budget/financing
• Patient evaluation	• Program evaluation

The treatment plan and the plan for the community are similar; both include the many facets of preparation, such as determining various methods, strategies, and costs of choosing a plan that will work best for the patient or community. The treatment and the program operation occur during the actual implementation of the plan. Payment for dental services is equated with program funding. Various methods of payment are often explored in both cases.

Evaluation of the treatment is similar to the program appraisal and should occur during the implementation and at the end of the treatment or operation.[5] This comparison should help the private practice hygienist become comfortable with the concepts of community program planning, implementation, and evaluation (see Chapter 5).

▨ GOVERNMENT'S ROLE IN PUBLIC HEALTH

Government Agencies

As a dental hygienist, you may contribute to the health of people in the community through participating in community health promotion activities. You may choose to present an educational presentation at a school or conduct a cancer screening at a facility for older residents (see Chapter 7). The more formal public health programs, however, generally fall under the aegis of the government. Both prevention and the delivery of services are concerns within the programs developed by government agencies.

The federal government's role in participating in dental health related activities falls under the jurisdiction of the **Department of Health and Human Services (DHHS).** *Healthy People 2010,* a publication of the DHHS, lists health objectives for the United States, including oral health, that need to be achieved by the year 2010 (see Chapter 4).

The Public Health Service (PHS) is one of four major agencies within the DHHS. The PHS promotes health standards, ensures that the highest level of health care is available for all citizens, and cooperates with other nations on health projects. There are eight operating agencies under the

Public Health Service (Fig. 1–2). Agencies that are of importance because they are involved in oral health programs include the following:

- Centers for Disease Control and Prevention (CDC)
- Health Resources and Services Administration (HRSA)
- National Institutes of Health (NIH), National Institute of Dental Research (NIDR)
- Agency for Healthcare Research and Quality (AHRQ)[7]

At the state level, public health agencies have been charged with the task of developing oral health programs within their state. These programs usually include educational programs for children under 18 years of age. Restorative and emergency services are often included through community clinics. Screening and data collection for needs assessments are also conducted at this level.

At the local level, dental programs vary throughout the nation. As a result of a decline in funding at all levels, there has been less involvement at this level in recent years and fewer data have been collected to determine needs.[8]

Core Functions of Public Health

Federal, state, and local programs have been charged to improve the health of the people through assessment, policy development, and assurance.

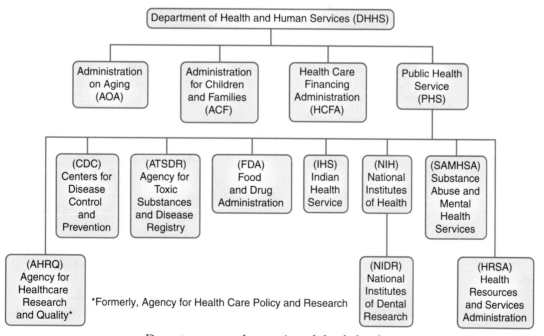

Figure 1–2. Departments and agencies of the federal government.

These core public health functions of **assessment, policy development,** and **assurance** were identified in an Institute of Medicine (IOM) report in 1988. This report states that the core public health functions were developed to protect and promote health, wellness, and the quality of life as well as to prevent disease, injury, disability, and death.[9] Figure 1–3 presents these core functions.

Assessment
- Every public health agency regularly and systematically collects, assembles, analyzes, and makes available information on the health of the community, including statistics on health status, community health needs, and epidemiologic and other studies of health problems. Not every agency is large enough to conduct these activities directly; intergovernmental and interagency cooperation is essential. Nevertheless, each agency bears the responsibility for seeing that the assessment function is fulfilled. This basic function of public health cannot be delegated.

Policy development
- Every public health agency exercises its responsibility to serve the public interest in the development of comprehensive public health policies by promoting use of the scientific knowledge base in decision-making about public health and by leading in developing public health policy. Agencies must take a strategic approach, developed on the basis of a positive appreciation for the democratic political process.

Assurance
- Public health agencies assure their constituents that services necessary to achieve agreed upon goals are provided, either by encouraging actions by other entities (private or public sector), by requiring such action through regulation, or by providing services directly.
- Each public health agency involves key policymakers and the general public in determining a set of high-priority personal and community-wide health services that governments will guarantee to every member of the community. This guarantee should include subsidization or direct provision of high-priority personal health services for people unable to afford them.

Figure 1–3. Core functions of public health agencies at all levels of government are assessment, policy development, and assurance. (Adapted from Institute of Medicine Committee for the Study of the Future of Public Health, Division of Health Care Services: A Vision of Public Health in America: An Attainable Ideal. Washington, DC, National Academy Press, 1998.)

Public health
- Prevents epidemics
- Protects against environmental hazards
- Prevents injuries
- Promotes and encourages healthy behaviors
- Responds to disasters and assists communities in recovery
- Assures the quality and accessibility of health services

Essential public health services
- Monitor health status to identify community health problems
- Diagnose and investigate health problems and health hazards in the community
- Inform, educate, and empower the public about health issues
- Mobilize community partnerships to identify and solve health problems
- Develop policies and plans to support individual and community health efforts
- Enforce laws and regulations that protect the public's health and ensure safety
- Link people to needed personal health services
- Assure a competent public health and personal health care work force
- Evaluate effectiveness, accessibility, and quality of personal and population-based health services
- Conduct research for new insight and innovative solutions to health problems

Figure 1–4. Essential public health services in the United States. (From Public Health in America. Washington, DC, Public Health Functions Steering Committee, 1994.)

The public health functions have been further delineated since the publication of the Institute of Medicine report. Through a consensus development process, a number of organizations and agencies produced a document entitled *Public Health in America*. This document lists essential public health services necessary to accomplish the core public health functions (Fig. 1–4). Successful provision of these services requires collaboration among private and public partners within the community and across various levels of government. These services are essential to achievement of healthy people in healthy communities.[10]

Building on the framework of the core public health functions and the essential public heath services, the Association of State and Territorial Dental Directors (ASTDD) developed guidelines for state oral health programs within state health departments (see Chapter 5). The core public health functions, the essential public health services, and the essential public health services for oral health provide guidance

for dental public health professionals working at national, state, and local levels.

FUTURE OF DENTAL PUBLIC HEALTH

What Needs to Be Done

Over the years, the number of dental public health programs at federal,
state, and local levels has declined as a result of tight budgets and di-
minishing resources. Dental disease persists as a public health problem
that can be alleviated and, possibly, eliminated. The knowledge exists,
but because of restraints and a lack of resources, this knowledge is not
being applied toward the goal of communities free from dental disease.
The ongoing need to emphasize the importance of oral health has never
been stronger. It is the responsibility of the dental health professionals to
emphasize the connection of oral health to people's general health to the
policymakers of our nation. Corbin and Marten's report[11] on the future
of dental health states that although oral health needs are documented,
oral health is given a low priority by health planners. The report emphasizes goals to meet for improved dental public health (see "Guiding
Principles").

Guiding Principles

Goals to Be Met to Improve Dental Public Health[11]

* Earn support from the public

* Earn support from the policymakers

* Earn support from program administrators

* Earn support from the dental community

* Ensure recruitment and professional development of dental public
  health personnel

* Ensure collaboration with colleagues

Going in the Right Direction

Although the dental profession must continue to seek legislation and
funding for health programs and to educate the public on the relationship of oral health to general health, the profession appears to be moving in the direction of success. A 1999 report by the CDC[12] lists the
10 most important public health accomplishments of the 20th century.
This list is encouraging and supportive to the efforts of all public health
professionals (see "Guiding Principles" on page 11).

Guiding Principles

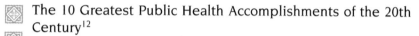

The 10 Greatest Public Health Accomplishments of the 20th Century[12]

- A significant decline in deaths from coronary heart disease and stroke as a result of behavior modification, a decrease in smoking, and early intervention programs

- The 1964 Surgeon General's acknowledgment of tobacco as a health hazard and resultant antismoking campaigns that have changed the public health perceptions about the habit

- Vaccination, which has helped to eradicate smallpox and to manage diseases such as measles, rubella, and tetanus

- Improved motor vehicle safety, with greater emphasis placed on personal responsibility for reducing motor vehicle–related fatalities caused by drinking and reckless driving

- Control of infectious diseases, which has been aided by improved water sanitation and better understanding of the science of microbiology

- Safer workplaces that have contributed to a higher standard of living and a 40% reduction in job-related injuries and fatalities

- Safer and healthier foods as a result of less microbial contamination as well as fortification of foods with supplements and vitamins

- Healthier mothers and babies, thanks to improved prenatal care and greater access to care

- Better access to family planning information and greater use of contraceptives, which has improved the socioeconomic status of United States citizens

- Fluoride in drinking water, which reaches 144 million people safely and is an inexpensive method of preventing tooth decay independent of a person's socioeconomic status

Dental hygienists play an important role in assessing and prioritizing dental health needs in the community. They have a responsibility to participate in the activities that will list community oral health practice as an important achievement in the 21st century. Social responsibility and the dental hygienist's commitment to the community are discussed in Chapter 8.

The dental hygienists who have chosen careers as state dental directors or public health educators contribute to the advancement of dental public health, but much more needs to be accomplished by all members of the dental hygiene profession. Through various roles, dental hygienists can affect the oral health of all people (Fig. 1–5).

Figure 1–5. Six roles of the dental hygienist.

> 1. Service Provider/Clinician
> 2. Health Educator/Wellness Promoter
> 3. Consultant/Resource Person
> 4. Consumer Advocate/Change Agent
> 5. Researcher
> 6. Administrator/Manager

SIX ROLES OF THE DENTAL HYGIENIST

Definition of Roles

The following roles of the dental hygienist demonstrate the various opportunities for the profession to be involved in improving people's health. Future chapters cover the knowledge and skills necessary to develop these roles. Chapter 2 describes the skills necessary to become actively involved at various levels and further describes career opportunities involving the six roles that the hygienist may play within the field of public health. Herein, as an introduction, are their definitions.

- **Service Provider/Clinician**. The dental hygienist assesses oral health conditions and develops a plan to manage oral diseases. Treatment is then provided.
- **Health Educator/Wellness Promoter**. Preventing disease and promoting oral health through the presentation of scientific information on topics such as fluoridation make this role crucial to the improvement and enhancement of oral health.
- **Consultant/Resource Person**. The dental hygienist is the liaison between the community and the dental profession. In this role, the dental hygienist determines the appropriate program or activity that will serve the needs of the community.
- **Consumer Advocate/Change Agent**. In this role, the dental hygienist must have the knowledge and skills to work legislatively to promote change and advance the health of the public through legislation, public policy, research, and science. As a consumer advocate, the dental hygienist represents individuals or large groups of consumers and informs them of quality services and products.
- **Researcher**. As a researcher, the dental hygienist determines which methods of prevention work best for the people served by the profession. This includes evaluating products and techniques and sharing the findings.
- **Administrator/Manager.** In both the private office and in the public health arena, the dental hygienist administers and manages programs. Within the administrator role, many functions of the other roles are required.

Common Goal in All Roles

The goal of dental public health is optimal oral health for all citizens and universal access to comprehensive dental care. To accomplish this goal, dental hygienists perform duties within the six roles listed. Both dentists and dental hygienists have entered the field of public health by accepting employment within programs that include health promotion, community disease prevention, and provision of dental care to selected groups of people.

Dentists become recognized specialists in the field of dental public health through specialty certification with the American Board of Dental Health. In most states, dental hygienists have no required formal or specialty education to work within this field in the community, although some have pursued advanced degrees in public health or community health. Further education prepares the dental hygienist to work with underserved populations who continually face barriers to health care. These barriers, such as inadequate geographic and financial access, pose challenges to the dental and dental hygiene profession.

In an attempt to reach underserved populations (see Chapter 2), some states are permitting less restrictive dental hygiene supervision for dental hygienists working in the community. In 1998, the California legislature recognized a new title, the Registered Dental Hygienist in Alternative Practice Settings (RDHAP). The purpose of the title is to qualify dental hygienists to practice community oral health with less supervision in underserved areas. The dental hygienist who has a concern for the improvement and protection of the oral health of the whole population can participate in community oral health practice at a level of personal choice.

Summary

An understanding of people's health includes learning the basic terminology to define health, public health, and dental public health. People's health is the health of the public living within a community, state, or nation. Identifying public health problems and solutions provides dental hygienists with the knowledge to explore this field of health further and a means by which they might become involved. The government's role in people's health is mentioned briefly as an introduction to the programs to be discussed in more detail in future chapters. Comparison of private practice to community oral health practice demonstrates the similarities and prepares dental hygienists for the planning, implementation, and evaluation phases that constitute public health programs. As health care providers, with many roles and responsibilities, dental hygienists have a calling and a duty to serve the community in which they live.

Applying Your Knowledge

1. Bring articles to class from the daily news or current magazines that present a public health issue, and discuss what the problem is and how it is being addressed. (Use the seven characteristics described in this chapter to evaluate the issue.)
2. Choose a government public health program and further investigate its purpose and success in accomplishing this purpose. (See Web sites for state oral health programs, Chapter 5.)
3. Choose one of the six roles of the dental hygienist and explain how dental hygienists improve the oral health of their community through this role.

Dental Hygiene Competencies

Reading the material within this chapter and participating in the activities of Applying Your Knowledge will contribute to the student's ability to demonstrate the following competencies:

Health Promotion and Disease Prevention
HP.1 Promote the values of oral health and general health and wellness to the public and organizations within and outside the profession.
HP.4 Identify individual and population risk factors, and develop strategies that promote health related quality of life.

References

1. Constitution of the World Health Organization. Geneva, World Health Organization, 1946, p 3.
2. Winslow CE: The untitled fields of public health. Mod Med 2:183, 1920.
3. Block LE: Dental public health: An overview. In Gluck GM, Morganstein WM (eds): Jong's Community Dental Health, 4th ed. St. Louis, Mosby–Year Book, 1998.
4. Knutson JW: What is public health? In Pelton WJ, Wisan JM (eds): Dentistry in Public Health, 2nd ed. Philadelphia, WB Saunders, 1955.
5. Burt BA, Ecklund SA: Dentistry, Dental Practice, and the Community, 4th ed. Philadelphia, WB Saunders, 1999.
6. Allukian M, Horowitz A: Effective community prevention programs for oral diseases. In Gluck GM, Morganstein WM (eds): Jong's Community Dental Health, 4th ed. St. Louis, Mosby–Year Book, 1998.
6a. Oral Health in America: A report of the Surgeon General. Rockville, Md, U.S. Department of Health and Human Services, National Institute of Dental and Craniofacial Research, National Institutes of Health, 2000.
7. Gluck GM, Morganstein WM: Jong's Community Dental Health, 4th ed (Appendix A). St. Louis, Mosby–Year Book, 1998.
8. Kuthy R, Odum JG: Local dental programs: A descriptive assessment of funding and activities. J Public Health Dent 48:36, 1988.
9. Institute of Medicine Committee for the Study of the Future of Public Health, Division of Health Care Services: A Vision of Public Health in America: An Attainable Ideal in the Future of Public Health. Washington, DC, National Academy Press, 1998.
10. Public Health in America. Washington, DC, Public Health Functions Steering Committee, 1994.
11. Corbin SB, Marten FR: Future of dental public health report—preparing dental public health to meet the challenges: Opportunities of the 21st century. J Public Health Dent 54:80, 1994.
12. American Dental Hygienists Association: Lifestyle, Public Health Top Ten. Access 13:7, 1999.

Careers in Public Health for the Dental Hygienist

Sharon Logue, RDH, MPH
Kathy Voigt Geurink, RDH, MA

OBJECTIVES

Upon completion of this chapter, the student will be able to:

◆ Explain public health career options for dental hygienists

◆ Differentiate between career options available independently and through community agencies

◆ Discuss public health careers as a means of addressing the problem of access to oral health care

◆ Define skills and educational requirements for various roles in public health

◆ Explain the relationship of private practice activities to public health activities

◆ Identify specific careers, categorized by the six roles of the dental hygienist

Key Terms

Alternative Practice	Follow-up/Referral	Social Marketing
Primary Prevention	Health Education	Technical Assistance
General Supervision	Networking	Legislative/Policy Changes
Shortage Areas		

Opening Statement

Career Possibilities

- *Public health hygienist at a local health department*
- *Statewide coordinator for a school-based fluoride mouth rinse program*
- *Dental hygienist at a Veterans Administration hospital*
- *Dental hygienist working with a state migrant farm worker program*
- *Dental hygienist at a state correctional facility*
- *State dental director in a state health department*
- *Dental hygienist with a university hospital department*
- *Dental health educator with a school system*
- *Dental hygienist on a dental sealant team*
- *Dental hygienist in the U.S. Public Health Service*
- *Dental hygienist contracting for service in a nursing home*
- *Consultant to a Head Start program*

COMMUNITY ORAL HEALTH PRACTICE AS A CAREER

Public health careers for dental hygienists run the gamut from high-level administrative posts to providing oral hygiene care for elderly residents in a nursing home or providing dental education for school-aged children. In the public health field, some dental hygienists have an associate's degree or certificate, a bachelor's, a master's, or a doctorate degree. Many dental hygienists with advanced degrees working in public health began their public health careers with the minimum level of education. They chose to continue their education as their interests developed, their challenges expanded, and their desire grew to do more for the oral health of their community. A career in community oral health practice offers a variety of rewarding experiences that tend to feed the desire to make a difference in the oral health of all people.

We have provided a career chapter in the beginning of this text in order to allow you to make a connection with the role you might play in performing the functions discussed in the successive chapters. In private practice, the individual patient is your focus; in public health, the community is your patient. Your responsibilities will advance beyond individual clinical care, although in many positions individual care still remains a very important duty. Public health takes you into the realm of program development, implementation, and evaluation and offers an opportunity to work with various populations, other professionals, agencies, financing mechanisms, and rules and regulations.

▓ FUTURE TRENDS FOR DENTAL HYGIENISTS IN PUBLIC HEALTH

The Problem of Access to Oral Health Care

In a national report entitled *Oral Health in America,* the Surgeon General reviewed the profound disparities among specific population groups in oral health status and access to dental care.[1] Dental disease has been a chronic problem among low-income populations.[2] Federal agencies and state governments are addressing these gaps in access to oral health care through legislation and policy development. Examples of some actions created through these processes are shown in "Guiding Principles" next.

Guiding Principles

Creating Access to Oral Health Care Through Legislation and Policy Development[2, 3]

- ◆ Allocating additional funds for dental services

- ◆ Expanding treatment for special populations

- ◆ Creating volunteers and donated dental services

- ◆ Providing service programs

- ◆ Additional dental benefits through existing public insurance programs

- ◆ Extending educational loans and loan forgiveness for dental professionals

- ◆ Creating tax credits for providers

- ◆ Forming career ladders for dental providers

- ◆ Increasing flexible licensure requirements

- ◆ Increasing the scope of the dental hygienist's duties

- ◆ Expanding coverage for provider services

Some of these developments may increase the demand for dental hygienists in community oral health practice.

Alternative Practice Settings

Public health settings are categorized as **alternative practice** settings (i.e., providing oral hygiene services outside the private office in a "nontraditional" setting). Examples of the setting might be a community clinic, a mobile van, a school, a hospital, or a nursing home (Figs. 2–1 and 2–2). The delivery of dental services offered in private practice does not reflect the need for services for those without means or without the capability of accessing care. In an alternative setting, dental care can be brought to people in need. Dental hygienists can provide preventive services in these settings, reaching large numbers of people who might not otherwise receive care.

Preventive services, or **primary prevention**, are more effective, less costly, and involve less technology than secondary or tertiary prevention (Fig. 2–3) (see page 20). Methods such as fluoride mouth rinse programs, nutritional counseling, dental health education to community groups, and oral hygiene services and instruction are at the primary level.

Figure 2–1. A dental hygienist is providing oral hygiene care to a resident of a nursing home.

Figure 2–2. *A*, A mobile dental van is used as an alternative practice setting. *B*, Inside treatment area, mobile dental van.

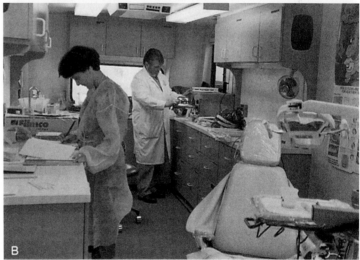

Often primary prevention strategies do not require a dentist.[4] Therefore, with less restrictive supervision, the dental hygienist can perform functions at this level and reach underserved populations.

Public Health Supervision

Regulatory Changes

Because of the need for services in places such as schools, nursing homes, and migrant health centers, dental hygienists are initiating oral health programs in these alternative settings. They are also filling

- **PRIMARY PREVENTION** prevents the disease before it occurs. This level includes health education, disease prevention, and health protection. (Dental prophylaxis, sealants, and water fluoridation are examples.)

- **SECONDARY PREVENTION** eliminates or reduces diseases in the early stages. (Restorations such as amalgams or composites are examples. This level requires more technology and is more costly than primary prevention.)

- **TERTIARY PREVENTION** limits disability from disease in later stages and requires rehabilitation and surgical procedures. (Dentures, implants, and bridge work are examples. This level is most costly and requires highly trained professionals to treat the disease.)

Figure 2–3. Levels of prevention.

positions beyond those connected with public health agencies. To create such positions, dental hygiene regulatory changes are being discussed and are now under way throughout the United States. Most states allow the dental hygienist to practice under **general supervision** (i.e., the dentist need not be on site but the patient must have been one of record or must have been seen by the dentist previously). Between 1991 and 1999, seven states passed laws to permit less restrictive dental hygiene supervision, allowing for dental hygienists to reach underserved populations. Figure 2–4 illustrates these states, including Colorado, which since 1987 has allowed unsupervised practice in all settings, and Washington, which since 1984 has allowed unsupervised practice in alternative settings, provided that the dental hygienist refers the patient to a dentist for further treatment.

In determining the necessity of regulatory changes, one must consider many factors, such as

1. The ratio of dentists to people.
2. The number of dentists and dental hygienists in the state.
3. The number of low-income adults and children who need dental care.

These factors contribute to defining dental health professional **shortage areas**. Statistics compiled from the 2000 Synopsis of State and Territorial Dental Health Programs provide information necessary in determining the available work force of dental professionals and of community health departments and clinics.[5] The work force numbers, compared with population size, are useful in determining professional shortage areas and the need for community oral health programs. Inadequate access to health care due to professional shortages and to geographic and financial barriers prevents people from attaining improved health status and improved

1999	**NEW MEXICO**	Dental hygienists practicing in a cooperative working relationship with a consulting dentist without general supervision may be certified "collaborative dental hygienist."
1998	**CALIFORNIA**	Registered dental hygienists in alternative practice (RDHAP) provide service in facilities and professional shortage areas with a prescription from a dentist or a physician.
1997	**OREGON**	Limited-access dental hygiene permit to treat patients in alternative settings; RDH must refer the patient annually to a licensed dentist available to treat the patient.
1997	**CONNECTICUT**	Pilot program to allow an RDH to practice in specific settings without supervision.
1995	**MAINE**	Public health supervision with permit to practice in specified alternative settings with a dentist who consults at the end of the project or annually but without general supervision.
1993	**NEW HAMPSHIRE**	Public health supervision with authorization of a dentist in an alternative setting; dentist reviews records annually.
1991	**MICHIGAN**	RDH permitted to treat the underserved, provided that the dentist is available for review and consultation.
1987	**COLORADO**	Unsupervised practice allowed in all settings.
1984	**WASHINGTON**	Unsupervised practice allowed in alternative settings, provided that the dental hygienist refers patient to a dentist for dental treatment and planning.

Figure 2–4. States permitting less restrictive dental hygiene supervision. (Data from Schroder K: States permitting unsupervised practice/less restrictive supervision. American Dental Hygienists Association, Division of Governmental Affairs [personal communication, 1998]. Reprinted in J Dent Hygiene 74:118, 2000.)

quality of life. The dental profession, in realizing the need for reaching these underserved populations, is initiating preventive programs conducted by dental hygienists in various states.

Public Health Supervision in Maine

In the state of Maine, data were collected and analyzed between May 1995, when the law allowed dental hygienists to practice without general supervision in alternative settings, and November 1998. Of 761 Registered Dental

Figure 2–5. Applicants for public health licensure in Maine.

Dental hygienists licensed in Maine	761
Dental hygienists granted public health licensure	38
Dental hygienists with an agency or a school	23
Dental hygienists initiating their own projects	15

Hygienists in Maine, 38 dental hygienists were granted public health licensure to conduct community oral health programs. Twenty-three (60%) of the dental hygienists were with a public health agency; 15 (40%) were applicants seeking board approval for programs in their own communities to address specific oral health needs (Fig. 2–5).[6] All nonagency dental hygienists were volunteers or unpaid. Although being a volunteer is an important concept in public health, the trend for dental hygienists to enter this arena will increase notably with the development of expanded payment mechanisms.

It is interesting that some dental hygienists, initially volunteers, have found creative ways to be reimbursed for working in alternative settings. Writing grants, seeking school board funds, collecting Medicaid payments through an accepted provider, or contracting with a facility, in states that allow it, are a few of the innovative reimbursement plans currently being used. With the less restrictive dental hygiene supervision and the increased number of dental hygienists seeking public health work, funding changes in the way of direct payment may be further explored in the future.

Dental hygienists in public health positions use a variety of skills in implementing community oral health programs that have positive effects on their communities. In this chapter, we further define the six roles of the dental hygienist (Fig. 2–6) as they apply to specific career options for the dental hygienist. Most public health jobs require a combination of skills defined in multiple roles. Positions held by dental hygienists working in public health are included to inspire and illustrate the variety of career possibilities.

▨ CAREERS IN DENTAL HYGIENE PUBLIC HEALTH

Service Provider/Clinician

In this familiar role, the public health dental hygienist provides clinical services to a targeted population, including assessment of oral health conditions and delivery of periodontal and preventive care. Often the population

Figure 2–6. Six roles of the dental hygienist.

1. Service Provider/Clinician
2. Health Educator/Wellness Promoter
3. Consultant/Resource Person
4. Consumer Advocate/Change Agent
5. Researcher
6. Administrator/Manager

Service Provider/Clinician

Dental
Hygienist
Mini-Profile

Name: Ginger Melton, RDH, BS

Position and Place of Employment:
Dental Hygienist
Portsmouth City Health
   Department
Portsmouth, Virginia

Qualifications and experience required for this position: Registered Dental Hygienist, Virginia Dental Hygiene License, at least 1 year of work experience; community education experience preferred.

Main dental hygiene role(s) fulfilled in this position: Service Provider/Clinician

Duties performed in this position: Provide dental health education, preventive dental services, and administrative services for the department. Serve schoolchildren and indigent adults. Provide oral hygiene services and education to children at school sites. Educate families about oral hygiene care.

Personal comment: As a public health dental hygienist, I face many challenges that are rewarding and motivating for me. In my clinical role, I provide much needed dental education, preventive services, and some administrative services. I am a "dental cheerleader" for a population that sees dental care as secondary. My challenge is to get the community to understand the importance of oral health and the prevention of disease.

served in a public health dental clinic has had limited access to dental care, has been excluded from dental benefits under employer insurance, and is often described as having lower socioeconomic status. Socioeconomic status includes factors such as income, education, and occupation. Populations of low socioeconomic status generally are at increased risk for dental disease.[7] These factors as well as different social and cultural values can influence utilization of dental services offered in public health clinics. Additional skills needed by the clinician include the ability to assess the perceived dental needs of the patient and to recognize the social and economic barriers to successful oral health outcomes. Examples of barriers to accessing dental services may include transportation problems, geographic distances, missed work hours, or lack of day care services for children.[8]

The clinician must know effective preventive strategies for populations who are at high risk for dental caries. Topical and systemic fluorides, dental sealants, and fluoride varnishes are preventive therapies to be considered for clinical care in public health settings. Health education classes and oral hygiene instructions need to be adapted for the community audience. The dental hygienist may require additional preparation, including health education courses that reinforce teaching methods. Public health dental programs address health problems that affect a large number of people and design solutions to work within the social and cultural contexts of communities. These programs influence individual and group behaviors and practices.

Alternative settings for dental clinics may be in fixed facilities or operatories at local health departments, in stationary school trailers, or in mobile dental vans that can be moved to various schools within a geographic area. Some states have school-based dental programs with dental teams who use portable dental equipment for placing dental sealants. Clinical dental hygiene positions are available in other community settings, including hospitals, nursing homes, and prison facilities. These locations offer the clinician additional challenges of complex medical histories and patients with physical or mental disabilities. Federal and state agencies have established clinical dental hygiene positions (e.g., the Indian Health Service, Community and Migrant Health Programs, military bases). In addition, clinical care programs in communities may be supported by nonprofit volunteer or religious organizations. In nonprofit and in publicly funded programs, these clinicians must be accountable with the most cost-effective way to provide quality dental services to the most people.

Public health dental hygienists may be asked to participate in the ongoing assessment of the prevalence of dental disease. This task is essential for public health program planning and evaluation. Clinical dental hygiene skills are used in conducting dental surveys and screenings for targeted populations. For example, a dental hygienist may be the coordinator who organizes a community-wide screening of school-aged children. The dental hygienist selects and uses appropriate supplies, portable equipment, and infection control procedures and communicates with school personnel and parents to create the screening schedules for schools. Knowledge of dental indices, data collection, and reporting of dental findings is essential.

In addition, with any screening program there must be a **follow-up/referral** component. Alerting the community to the problems discovered is part of the assessment; however, without the plan for action, the collection and presentation of data are ineffective. The plan for action includes a system to provide prevention and treatment for the documented needs.

Educational requirements for a public health clinical position may vary from an associate's degree to a bachelor's degree. If the public health job requires more administrative or consulting skills (see later), an employer may require more work experience or a master's degree.

Health Educator/Wellness Promoter

As in private practice, an important role of the public health dental hygienist is that of health educator. **Health education** is the process in which the client is encouraged to become responsible for personal oral

Educator/Wellness Promoter

Dental
Hygienist
Mini-Profile

Name: Leonor Ramos, RDH

Position and Place of Employment:
Hospital Dentistry Dental Hygienist
Department of Defense, United States Air Force
Wilford Hall Medical Center
Lackland Air Force Base, Texas

Qualifications and experience required for this position: Registered Dental Hygienist, graduated from an accredited school of dental hygiene. Broad-based knowledge of complex medical and pathologic conditions and their impact on overall health. Experienced in providing appropriate clinical techniques and instructions for oral care and able to perform complex functions that differ with the needs of each medically compromised patient. Exceptional judgment, organizational skills, and leadership qualities preferred.

Main dental hygiene role(s) fulfilled in this position: Educator, Clinician

Duties performed in this position:

Educator: Educate hospitalized patients on oral hygiene care, provide numerous in-service presentations to various medical professionals on the oral management of medically compromised patients, present continuing education programs in this area, supervise dental hygiene students on a hospital rotation, provide yearly lectures on oral management of cancer patients to dental hygiene students, coordinate annual National Dental Hygiene Month Symposium for federally employed dental hygienists, organize continuing education programs for military trained prophylaxis technicians and dental hygienists at this installation (Lackland Air Force Base) through Preventive Dentistry Committee.

Clinician: Provide preoperative and postoperative preventive oral care for urgent hospitalized surgical patients who require dental clearance before their surgery. Included are patients receiving organ transplants, bone marrow transplants, and major orthopedic joint replacements; chronically ill patients; patients with hematologic disorders; patients with poorly controlled diabetes; patients in intensive critical care units; and terminally ill patients who need palliative oral care.

Personal comment: My experience in public health began when I trained as a preventive dentistry technician while on active duty with the Air Force. Eventually, I left active duty in order to pursue my license as a dental hygienist at the University of Texas Health Science Center in San Antonio. At the same time, as an Air Force reservist I

Profile continued on following page

Educator/Wellness Promoter Continued

trained to be an aeromedical technician. This combination of medical and dental training provided me with the ideal background to be selected for a new position at Wilford Hall in the field of hospital dentistry. Now in the 27th year of my public health career, I continue to hold that position, which is both one-of-a-kind and unique to the military. Recently, I had the opportunity to participate in the development of a publication for health care professionals, which I initiated through the Texas Cancer Council. The booklet, *Oral Health in Cancer Therapy*, is available through the Oral Health Education Foundation, Inc., P.O. Box 396, Fairburn, GA 30213. I now provide training to federally employed nurses entering the field of oncology, as well as to dental hygiene students, on the oral management of cancer patients.

health and is informed of scientifically based methods for preventing dental diseases. Beyond dental health education, though, is the promotion of total wellness. The community dental health educator must reinforce the relationship of oral health to total health.

Early childhood caries may be the result of infant feeding practices that are related to nutritional issues. Improved dietary habits by adults may mean less risk of dental decay and less risk of other chronic diseases. The dental hygienist working at the community level always needs to consider the larger picture of wellness in creating education programs. For example, current research indicates a possible relationship between periodontal health, cardiovascular health, incidence of premature births, and diabetes. Programs planned to intervene in these chronic diseases must be expanded to include oral health education.[9]

The team approach is always essential in public health. Dental health educators can participate in **networking** with other health professionals (i.e., they can share information about a common population). School nurses may have a unique perspective on the dental needs of schoolchildren, and sharing this information is helpful in program planning. Networking means that health statistics, resources for educational materials, and general community information are exchanged among dentists, physicians, dental hygienists, nurses, and nutritionists. As noted at a symposium (Children, Our Future) in 1998,[10] "the lack of integration of oral health into overall health adds a significant barrier to improving children's health outcomes." All health professionals must understand the impact of oral disease on systemic health. Effective networking among dental hygienists and other health professionals increases the awareness and importance of the relationship of oral health to general health. Community education, therefore, can be designed to include several health messages for a target group. This team approach is comprehensive and cost-effective.

Public health education programs have built upon the success of commercial marketing techniques by means of **social marketing** to promote the adoption of a behavior to improve health. Social marketing refers to using the effective advertising tools from commercial marketing to influence a valued health behavior change. Dental hygienists can use social marketing concepts to develop a public awareness campaign, to create educational materials, or to improve dental services.

An effective health educator researches the target population to identify the community's needs and concerns about dental health. A town forum or smaller focus groups may be organized to learn about the community's ideas on dental issues. Dental hygienists must study and understand the community in order to develop the appropriate message; they then monitor health education programs and, finally, readjust programs to meet changing trends. Mass media, the means of communication that reaches large numbers of people, can be a marketing tool. Skills in writing newspaper or newsletter articles and developing television and radio public service announcements can be valuable assets in a public health education position. Even the development of a dental health Web site can be a job responsibility.

Dental health educators may work statewide on preventive programs or may work with smaller, targeted populations at the county or community level. Examples of oral health education programs include:

- ◆ A spit tobacco intervention program related to prevention of oral cancer
- ◆ Promotion of dental sealants for schoolchildren
- ◆ Education about prevention of early childhood caries (baby bottle tooth decay) in cooperation with public health nutritionists
- ◆ A dental poster contest for third-graders
- ◆ Adoption of fluoridation in a community
- ◆ Promotion of mouth guards for athletes in a school district.

The months of February (National Children's Dental Health Month) and October (Dental Hygiene Month) provide excellent opportunities for oral health educational activities.

The successful dental health education program is planned to target a specific dental concern or a need identified in a population. Dental health educators in the community need organizational skills, current scientific knowledge, excellent communication skills, creativity, and flexibility to meet the challenges of community health improvement (see Chapter 7). Educational requirements for health educator positions may vary from a 2-year degree to a graduate degree, depending on specific job requirements.

Consultant/Resource Person

A public health dental hygienist may be asked to be a resource person for dental information and provide **technical assistance** at the local, state, or federal level. Technical assistance refers to the use of professional skills and a knowledge base to provide guidance to nondental

Consultant/Resource Person

Name: JoAnn W. Wells, RDH, BS

Position and Place of Employment:
Human Services Program
  Coordinator
Virginia Department of Health
Division of Dental Health
Richmond, Virginia

Qualifications and experience required for this position: Undergraduate degree in dental hygiene. Preferred: master's degree in an educationally related area or with a strong emphasis in health education and at least 1 year of work experience.

Main dental hygiene role(s) fulfilled in this position: Consultant/ Resource Person

Duties performed in this position: Act as a consultant for Head Start Programs, Department of Health and Human Services, Region III. Plan and present workshops with Head Start health coordinators, teachers and parents on fluoride supplements, fluoride dosage schedule, use and handling of toothbrushes in the classroom setting, amount of toothpaste used by children, first aid in dental emergencies, healthy snacking, and basic dental health facts. As a resource person, assist in developing and dispursing educational materials, provide training workshops through the Department of Education for school nurses, school administrators, and teachers. Provide dental resources to other health care providers, nutritionists, and nursing staff at local health departments.

Personal comment: My concern is for the dental health of children and the educational achievement of young people. The recognition that education and health are intertwined has resulted in considerable interest in school health programs that engage the entire community. My experience with school administrators, school nurses, school teachers, parents, and caregivers is to focus on the child's oral health to achieve a common vision.

community members interested in developing preventive programs. In this role, the dental hygienist acts as a consultant to community agencies, schools, or other health professions on dental issues. Oral health education for persons who will deliver the dental message to other adults and children are examples of "train the trainer" activities. Oral health education can be targeted to Head Start Program, nursing home, and day care staffs; parent organizations; schoolteachers; coaches; school nurses; and nutritionists.

Another example of the resource/consultant role might involve representing the dental profession on local committees, such as the American Cancer Society, the American Heart Association, Head Start Health Advisory committees, local health partnership coalitions, and dental professional organizations. Committee options are unlimited. On a regional level, dental hygienists can be employed part time to be consultants and to review Head Start programs for compliance with program standards. State public health programs that monitor community water fluoridation may have dental hygienists who provide technical assistance to water engineers or to community leaders initiating a council vote on fluoridation. A school system considering starting a school-based fluoride mouth rinse program may ask for supportive testimony at a school board meeting from a dental hygienist.

As resource persons, dental hygienists can help guide the public on the appropriateness of available dental health educational materials. Given the existence of many information clearinghouses, the dental hygienist needs organizational skills to maintain current directories of dental resources. The Maternal and Child Health National Oral Health Clearinghouse is an example of a directory with dental educational materials appropriate for many community preventive programs. Public health dental programs must always be cost-effective, and national clearinghouses may often be good sources of quality materials at reasonable prices.

With communication technology constantly changing, knowledge of current dental Web sites for references is essential in this role. Web sites are a resource not only for professionals but also for consumers at all income levels who are gaining access to this form of communication. A dental hygienist can provide technical assistance by

1. Creating a Web page containing information on oral health.
2. Maintaining a lending library of dental brochures, videotapes, and educational displays available to the public.
3. Developing culturally appropriate educational materials to meet the needs of community groups.

Dental schools and dental hygiene education programs may request guest lectures on community oral health from a resource person. Student interactions with public health staff can only add to an increased understanding of public health policies and their positive impact on society. A dental hygienist may coordinate an extramural public health rotation for dental hygiene students and get them involved in health promotion activities. Educational requirements for a consultant/resource person may range from a bachelor's degree to a master's degree.

Consumer Advocate/Change Agent

With the community considered to be a "patient," the public health dental hygienist assesses the dental needs and concerns of the population. After exploring the available dental resources, the dental hygienist identifies

Consumer Advocate/Change Agent

Name: Carol Marchisotto Reid, RDH, BS

Position and Place of Employment:
Public Health Dental Hygienist
Rockingham County Department of Health
North Carolina Department of Health and Human Services
Division of Public Health
Oral Health Section
Wentworth, North Carolina

Qualifications and experience required for this position: Undergraduate degree in dental hygiene. Preferred: master's degree in an educationally related area or with a strong emphasis in health education and at least 1 year of work experience.

Main dental hygiene role(s) fulfilled in this position: Consumer Advocate/Change Agent

Duties performed in this position: Assessing community needs, informing professionals and community leaders of people's needs within the community, planning and implementing programs to produce a positive change, and improving the oral health of the citizens. I participated in the following programs: health education and promotion, community water fluoridation, school weekly fluoride mouth rinse programs, sealants and fluoride varnish programs, and screening with referral and follow-up.

Personal comment: I was a laboratory technician and a dental assistant before entering the field of dental hygiene. My strong desire to help people improve their oral health led me to practice community oral health. As a public health dental hygienist, I help prevent dental disease and to reduce the pain and suffering of persons living in my community. I am able to work at multiple levels with schools, health departments, community organizations, and the media to reach a majority of persons of all ages and backgrounds. Learning about the gap in access to care for the indigent population, I was instrumental in starting a new county dental clinic to serve the needs of children and adults receiving Medicaid. I know prevention and treatment together are a winning combination for the improvement of oral health for underserved populations.

any "gaps" in oral health services for specific populations. A gap refers to the inability of a group of individuals to receive, or have access to, oral health services. For example, an indigent group of older adults may lack finances to obtain dental care. The dental hygienist might represent these individuals in seeking community resources and in developing special

programs. Once consumer issues are brought to the attention of local media or powerful citizens, changes can occur and problems can be solved.
The consumer advocate sees problems related to achieving optimal oral
health and attempts to develop a solution.

As a dental professional, the hygienist can be a leader for the consumer
and can be asked to be a vocal advocate for oral health. Dental hygienists
who serve on state dental boards are evaluating skills of recent graduates,
thus protecting the public and acting as a consumer advocate. The role of
consumer advocate/change agent may not be a full-time position but may
be part of another role in the dental hygiene profession. A request for expert testimony on dental issues might come from state legislative bodies or
boards of health. In this role, the dental hygienist is working to advance
the health of the public through **legislative** and public **policy changes**.

Legislative activity to change dental hygiene supervision laws is a task
of the dental hygienist in the role of change agent. The American Dental
Hygienists' Association cites restrictive supervision laws for dental hygienists as a barrier to access for oral health care. Dental hygienists working under *direct supervision* (i.e., a dentist must be physically present
during procedures performed by a hygienist) is limited in performing preventive services for segments of the population who do not have access to
regular oral health care, such as the poor, elderly, and disabled. Through
the role of change agent/consumer advocate, dental hygienists have
changed supervision from *direct* to *general* in many states. As a result of
legislative involvement by dental hygienists in California, certification of
the Registered Dental Hygienist in Alternative Practice (RDHAP) was initiated in 1998. The RDHAP is a licensed dental hygienist who provides
unsupervised dental hygiene services in settings such as schools or institutions as prescribed by a dentist or physician.[11]

Dental hygienists who become consumer advocates/change agents may
have several years of experience in their profession and have the ability to
visualize the "big picture." A specific educational degree beyond being a
Registered Dental Hygienist may not be needed in this role. An effective
consumer advocate/change agent is knowledgeable, confident, and eager
for all citizens to have optimal oral health.

Researcher

As a researcher, a dental hygienist uses scientific methods and knowledge
to identify and pursue a specific area of interest (see Chapter 6 for a discussion of the scientific method used in research). Dental hygienists employed in the research arena work in settings that vary from state health
departments to universities to private industry.

In a state health department dental program, the epidemiology of
dental diseases is a likely area of interest. Knowledge of dental indices to
survey the prevalence of dental diseases is required, and biostatistical

Researcher

Name: Kathy Phipps, RDH, MPH, DrPH

Position and Place of Employment:
Associate Professor, School of Dentistry
Research Associate Professor, School of Medicine
Oregon Health Sciences University
Portland, Oregon

Qualifications and experience required for this position: Doctoral degree with experience in research; postdoctoral research fellowship recommended. With research experience, candidate may be in the process of doctoral degree completion.

Main dental hygiene role(s) fulfilled in this position: Researcher

Duties performed in this position: Research is concerned with epidemiology, or the study of disease trends in populations. With an RDH background, oral epidemiology is the area of research that is emphasized. For example, the present researcher is studying the impact of fluoride on skeletal health (osteoporosis).

Assisting local, state, and federal agencies in tracking the oral health status of people in their jurisdictions is also a function of the position.

Research interests may be expanded from dentistry to medicine. This researcher is a co-investigator for a major 7-year research project looking at risk factors for osteoporosis, cardiovascular disease, and prostate cancer in older men.

Primary duties of the epidemiology aspect include writing grant proposals, developing research protocols, analyzing research data, and writing manuscripts. Research assistants actually work with the study participants and collect the data.

Personal comment: I am a graduate of the dental hygiene program at Oregon Health Sciences University with a bachelor of science degree in Dental Hygiene. At the same time, I also attended classes at Portland State University and received a bachelor of science degree in general science with an emphasis in public health studies.

After receiving my bachelor degrees, I practiced dental hygiene for about 1 year. I then applied to graduate school and received a scholarship to attend the Program in Dental Public Health, School of Public Health at the University of Michigan. My emphasis during the master's program was in health care administration. I returned to the state of Oregon and worked as a health administrator and social service manager for an agency serving senior citizens.

Researcher *Continued*

I was away from dentistry for about 6 years and decided that it was time to return to the field. I applied for and received funding to complete my doctoral degree at the University of Michigan. I became interested in fluoride and started doing my research on fluoride and osteoporosis while still in graduate school.

Since that time, I have had three research projects funded by the National Institute of Dental and Craniofacial Research. The results of these projects have been published in the *Journal of Dental Research* and the *British Medical Journal*.

Although research may not sound glamorous or exciting, it has given me an opportunity to experience many different aspects of life. For example, I have done research in Russia and remote villages in Alaska, I have made presentations to dentists and hygienists in both the United States and the United Kingdom, and I am on several advisory panels for the National Institutes of Health and the Centers for Disease Control and Prevention.

skills for analyzing data is important. Funding for state dental programs is becoming difficult to maintain, given the trend toward government downsizing in some states. Being accountable for public funds is an essential part of program evaluation. Dental data must be continually gathered to evaluate and demonstrate the effectiveness of public health programs in improving oral health and reducing barriers to oral health care.

In a research position, the dental hygienist coordinates a statewide needs assessment. For a dental survey of this size, the dental hygienist must select a sample of appropriate size across the state and obtain permission to examine a specific population. If an oral health needs assessment involves the caries rates for children, the researcher may work through the school system to arrange for the children to be examined. Dental examiners are trained to use the dental indices through a calibration exercise to ensure that valid data have been obtained by the survey. Ultimately, the dental data analysis is important for future public health program planning. Epidemiologic research is crucial in maintaining existing oral health programs or in initiating new ones.

Research positions are available at many university or dental school settings. For example, a dental hygienist might be hired to participate in a periodontal research project to study the effectiveness of a new antimicrobial product, a microbiology department might seek dental hygienists as research associates, or a dental hygienist at a Veterans' Affairs hospital might study therapeutic procedures for patients with head and neck cancer.

Certainly, dental product companies have ongoing research to scientifically determine the effectiveness of new methods and products to prevent and treat oral diseases. A dental hygienist working as a researcher has an appropriate background in basic science and dental science to join a research team. Dental hygienists choosing research positions may work part time as a researcher, with the remainder of the job description being one of the previously discussed roles. Educational requirements for research positions may require a bachelor's degree. The specific background needed for research positions varies with the employer.

Administrator/Manager

The expanded coordination needed for community-wide oral health programs creates the need for a dental hygienist to be an administrator/manager. In this role, the hygienist is an initiator who develops, organizes, and manages oral health programs to meet the needs of targeted

Administrator/Manager

Dental Hygienist Mini-Profile

Name:
Kathleen Mangskau RDH, MPA

Position and Place of Employment:
Director, Oral Health Program
North Dakota Department of
    Health
Department 301
600 E Boulevard Avenue
Bismarck, North Dakota

Qualifications and experience required for this position: Registered Dental Hygienist with a bachelor's degree in dental hygiene, business administration, public administration, or related field and 2 years of experience in the dental hygiene field.

Main dental hygiene role(s) fulfilled in this position: Administrator (primary); Change Agent, Consultant, and Educator (secondary). Position also offers opportunities for research and clinical responsibilities.

Duties performed in this position: Planning, directing, and evaluating a statewide oral health program in oral disease prevention and health promotion. Essential duties include planning and evaluation, management, education, consultation, policymaking, fiscal control, and supervision (see Fig. 2–7).

Personal comment: As a clinical dental hygienist, I was the individual who often volunteered to lead community projects and provide community oral health education. Although I did not realize it early in my career, visioning and management and organizational skills were my strengths. I also like change, and community oral health provides new opportunities for growth almost every day in my career.

JOB DESCRIPTION
ORAL HEALTH PROGRAM DIRECTOR
NORTH DAKOTA DEPARTMENT OF HEALTH

DIVISION: Maternal & Child Health
LOCATION: Judicial Wing, State Capitol   EMPLOYEE:
REPORTS TO: Maternal and Child Health Division Director

SUMMARY: The Dental Health Program Director is responsible for planning, developing, directing, and evaluating a statewide dental health program in oral disease prevention/health promotion according to the long-term goals of the department and the delegated duties in the Division of Maternal and Child Health.

ESSENTIAL DUTIES AND RESPONSIBILITIES include the following. Other duties may be assigned.

Planning and evaluation
- Develops Dental Health Program goals, objectives, and work plans.
- Conducts community and statewide assessment of dental health and dental health–related problems and resources to determine current needs:
    a. Plans and conducts surveys. Analyzes and disseminates results.
    b. Uses secondary data.
    c. Directs special projects in dental health and prepares and analyzes reports of findings.
- Monitors and evaluates oral health prevention projects.

Management
- Uses data to document, monitor, and evaluate dental health services, costs, and outcomes
- Supervises application of and implementation of and contract performance under state and federal grant programs.
- Analyzes and summarizes program data.
- Prepares progress, quarterly, annual, and other administrative reports.
- Develops administrative and operational relationships with other state and local health, human services, and education units.
- Recommends staffing needs to division director.

Education
- Interprets and disseminates current scientific information on oral health prevention and treatment to professionals in health and human service agencies, educational institutions, and the general public.
- Develops, updates, and evaluates dental health education materials for use in health agency programs.
- Arranges, plans, and conducts in-service and training programs for program staff, health professionals, educators, volunteers, and the public.
- Prepares monthly program communication to dental health staff.
- Participates in professional development activities (reading journals, attending professional meetings, etc.)

Consultation
- Provides oral health consultation and technical assistance to administrators, policymakers, other dental personnel and professionals in the health agencies, other human service professionals in related agencies, and educators in academic institutions.

Figure 2–7. Sample of typical job description for oral health program director.

Illustration continued on following page

Figure 2–7. *Continued*

Policymaking
- Establishes and revises policies and procedures for the Dental Health Program in compliance with Health department policies and federal rules, regulations, and guidelines.
- Advises senior policymakers and administrators on dental health related issues.
- Reviews and comments on proposed federal or state laws, regulations, standards, and guidelines being promulgated by legislators or regulatory agencies.
- Provides leadership and advocacy for oral health issues.

Fiscal control
- Prepares and controls the operating budget for the Dental Health Program.
- Oversees approval of dental health special initiative grants to local entities.
- Prepares grant proposals and contracts to obtain external funding and technical assistance to evaluate and expand dental health services.

Supervision
- Supervises and evaluates program administrative support staff.
- Supervises and evaluates regional dental health consultants.
- Recruits, orients, trains, supervises, and evaluates work performance of contract staff and volunteers for special projects.

groups of people. Planning skills may be required for local, state, or federal oral health programs. If the oral health program is implemented for a large population or within a large geographic area, supervision of other professional and technical staff may be required.

The type of oral health program managed depends on the needs of the population. For example, a hygienist may manage a statewide school-based fluoride mouth rinse program funded from state revenues or from a federal grant. In this position, the dental hygienist needs the following:

1. Knowledge of how systemic and topical fluorides work to prevent dental caries.
2. Good communication skills to establish a working relationship with school superintendents, principals, and teachers.
3. Organizational skills to plan a budget, to order supplies, and to keep records.
4. Knowledge of evaluation procedures to account for the cost versus the program effectiveness.

To assess the dental caries rate among participating schoolchildren, one ideally conducts a dental survey before and after initiating this preventive program. Writing skills are important for summarizing survey results and program successes and for soliciting for additional grant funds.

An administrator or manager may often have additional roles, as previously discussed. The administrator may be required to provide some consulting, to become an advocate for changing public policy, or to be involved with social marketing for a new oral health initiative. Educational requirements of this administrative role are usually several years of experience and a bachelor's or master's degree in a related field, such as public health or health administration (Fig. 2–7).

Summary

Various career options exist for dental hygienists in the public health arena. The public health career options offer many challenges and opportunities for the dental hygienist to become actively involved in providing optimal oral health for the community. The trend of less restrictive dental hygiene regulation in order to facilitate the dental hygienist's desire to provide preventive treatment to underserved populations is explored. Data collected on population numbers related to dental manpower and community programs are mentioned and can be located at the Web site for the Association of State and Territorial Dental Directors.

Public health career options and public health positions for dental hygienists are available in a variety of settings. Within the primary setting of your dental hygiene career, you may choose to develop skills to work as a clinician, educator, researcher, consultant, consumer advocate, or administrator. The skills and education necessary to fulfill these roles have been delineated in the chapter.

APPLYING YOUR KNOWLEDGE

1. Check with your state health department to determine whether public health or community dental hygiene positions are available in your community. Obtain a job description and evaluate the skills needed for this position using the six roles described in the chapter.
2. Research all available dental resources in your community for older adults who are unable to afford or travel to private dental offices. Whom would you contact to find out the location of these dental services? Write a job description for yourself to treat elderly residents unable to have access to care in private offices.
3. Review dental supervision laws in your state, and determine whether there is a need for change. Which populations might benefit from a change? How might you be involved in initiating a change?
4. Participate in a community rotation/service project that is considered an alternative practice setting.

Dental Hygiene Competencies

Reading the material in this chapter and participating in the activities of Applying Your Knowledge will contribute to the student's ability to demonstrate the following competencies:

Core Competencies
C.8 Communicate effectively with individuals and groups from diverse populations verbally and in writing.

Community Involvement
CM.3 Provide community oral health services in a variety of settings.

Professional Growth and Development
PGD.1 Identify alternative career options within health care, industry, education, and research, and evaluate the feasibility of pursuing dental hygiene opportunities.
PGD.2 Develop management and marketing strategies to be used in nontraditional health care settings.
PGD.3 Access professional and social networks and resources to assist entrepreneurial initiative.

References

1. Oral Health in America: A Report of the Surgeon General. Rockville, Md, U.S. Department of Health and Human Services, National Institute of Dental and Craniofacial Research, National Institutes of Health, 2000.
2. Oral Health: Dental Disease Is a Chronic Problem Among Low-Income Populations. Washington, DC, U.S. General Accounting Office, 2000.
3. State of the States: Overview of 1999 State Legislation on Access to Oral Health. Washington, DC, Center for Policy Alternatives, 1999.
4. Warren RC: Oral Health for All: Policy for Available, Accessible and Acceptable Care. Washington, DC, Center for Policy Alternatives, 1999.
5. Synopsis of State and Territorial Dental Public Health Programs: Association of State and Territorial Dental Directors (ASTDD) Home Page, 2000. *http://www.astdd.org.*
6. Beaulieu E: Dental Hygiene public health supervision changes in Maine law. J Dent Hyg 74:117, 2000.
7. Capilouto E: Improving the oral health of at-risk children. J Health Care Poor Underserved 2:132–145, 1991.
8. Brick P: Working in public health. Access 7:12–16, 1993.
9. Berthold M: Profiles in public health: Dental hygienists reach out. Access 12:13–21, 1998.
10. Mouradian WE: Introduction and Overview of Children's Oral Health: A forgotten area. Symposium: Children, Our Future. Seattle, 1998.
11. American Dental Hygienists Association, Division of Governmental Affairs, Stateline. Access 12:32–33, 2000.

Assessment in the Community

Jane E.M. Steffensen, RDH, MPH, CHES, BS

OBJECTIVES

Upon completion of this chapter, the student will be able to:

◆ Explain the importance of assessment as a core public health function

◆ Describe the roles of public health professionals in assessment

◆ Discuss the basic terms, concepts, and characteristics of epidemiology

◆ Describe the conceptual models that illustrate the determinants of health

◆ Identify the determinants of health that affect the health of individuals and communities

◆ Identify the specific stages of a planning cycle

◆ Discuss a community oral health improvement process

◆ Describe the main steps followed and key activities undertaken in a community oral health assessment

◆ Compare and contrast the different methods of data collection that can be used in community health assessments

Key Terms

Assessment

Epidemiology

Host Factors

Agent Factors

Environmental Factors

Determinants of Health

Mandala of Health

Systematic Approach to
Health Improvement

Planning Cycle

Assess

Plan

Implement

Evaluate

Community Oral Health
Improvement Process

Community Oral Health
Assessment

Community Profile

Data Collection

Quantitative Data

Qualitative Data

Opening Statement

National Leading Health Indicators

Indicators	Related Statistics*
◆ *Physical activity*	◆ *More than 60% of adults are not physically active on a regular basis*
◆ *Overweight and obesity*	◆ *54% of adults are overweight*
◆ *Tobacco use*	◆ *26% of men over 18 smoke*
◆ *Substance abuse*	◆ *14,843 deaths per year from drug-induced causes*
◆ *Mental health*	◆ *31.8 million office visits per year for mental disorders*
◆ *Injury and violence*	◆ *146,400 deaths per year due to injuries*
◆ *Environmental quality*	◆ *50,000 to 120,000 premature deaths per year associated with exposure to air pollutants*
◆ *Immunizations*	◆ *81% of population vaccinated against diphtheria*
◆ *Responsible sexual behavior*	◆ *13,426 deaths per year from AIDS/HIV[†] infection*
◆ *Access to personal health care*	◆ *14% of children younger than 18 years of age have no health insurance*

*Statistics 1996–1998 from *http://www.cdc.gov* (accessed September 2000).
[†]AIDS, acquired immunodeficiency syndrome; HIV, human immunodeficiency virus.

▩ PUBLIC HEALTH PRACTICE

Professional work in community health is dynamic because the environment changes continuously. Community health is affected by social, demographic, political, economic, and technologic changes. In this milieu, public health practitioners perform a broad array of duties focused on entire populations, with the overarching goal that people are healthy and live in healthy communities.[1, 2] The mission of public health is to "fulfill society's interest in assuring the conditions in which people can be healthy."[3, 4] Public health carries out this mission through organized, interdisciplinary efforts that address health problems in communities. Its mission is achieved through the application of health promotion and disease prevention and control efforts designed to improve health and enhance quality of life.[1, 2]

Public health services incorporate the roles of a myriad of public health professionals in various sectors and from diverse disciplines that form the public health work force in the United States.[1, 2] Public health professionals belong to many professional disciplines, including health promotion, environmental health, administration, and epidemiology.[5] Public health professionals have expertise in diverse public health practices.[1, 2] Education and training guidelines have been developed to extend capacity and to ensure that current and future public health professionals have expertise in key public health services.[5]

Successful provision of public health services requires collaboration among private and public partners within a given community and across various levels of government. To fulfill these responsibilities, partnerships must include private, voluntary, and public agencies or organizations involved in health, mental health, substance abuse, environmental health protection, and public health.[6] Examples of community organizations and participants that can form key partnerships to improve health in communities are presented in the Appendix C.

▩ ASSESSMENT: A CORE PUBLIC HEALTH FUNCTION

The contemporary principles of public health practice and science have been highlighted in *The Future of Public Health* report, which focuses attention on the discipline of public health.[3] This report, published by the Institute of Medicine (IOM), details past contributions and identifies future challenges to public health. It outlines recommendations to improve the nation's public health system and to ensure universal access to necessary public health services.

The IOM report specifies three core public health functions that shape the basic practice of public health at the state and local level.[3] State health agencies and local health departments must perform these functions in order to protect and promote health, wellness, and quality of life as well as to prevent disease, injury, disability, and death. These functions (as noted in Chapter 1) are (1) assessment, (2) policy development, and (3) assurance.[3] This chapter emphasizes the core public health function of assessment in the community.

The IOM report calls for public health agencies to promote, to facilitate, and—when necessary and appropriate—to perform community health assessments and to monitor change in key measures to evaluate performance. **Assessment** is defined as the regular and systematic collection, assemblage, analysis, and communication on the health of the community.[3] The IOM report states that assessment includes statistics on health status, community health needs, and epidemiologic and other studies of health problems.[3]

▨ ROLES OF PUBLIC HEALTH PROFESSIONALS IN ASSESSMENT

The effective use of information is crucial to ensure that healthy children and adults are living in healthy communities. As societies change in the 21st century new technologies will influence the capacity and ability to generate and collect a vast amount of information.[1, 2] Therefore, public health practitioners must have skills in collecting, analyzing, and using data and information.[5] It is essential for public health professionals to[5, 7]:

- Work with communities to form partnerships
- Gather health-related data
- Identify health issues and resources
- Determine priority health concerns
- Implement solutions to address community health problems
- Utilize data and evaluate outcomes of public health policies and interventions[8]

Future public health dental hygienists are likely to become more involved in community oral health assessments.[9, 10] As agencies and organizations take on greater responsibility in conducting periodic assessments, public health dental hygienists are expected to evaluate assets, needs, problems, and resources of the populations they serve in the community. Dental public health professionals within local and state health agencies are likely to be responsible for community oral health assessment.[9] Essential public health services for oral health were developed to describe community oral health assessment (see Chapter 5 and "Guiding Principles," next page).

Guiding Principles

Essential Public Health Services for Oral Health Related to Assessment[9]

◆ Assessment of oral health status and needs so that problems can be identified and addressed

◆ Analysis of determinants of identified oral health needs, including resources

◆ Assessment of the fluoridation status of water systems and other sources of fluoride

◆ Implementation of an oral health surveillance system to identify, investigate, and monitor oral health problems and health hazards

◆ Evaluation of effectiveness, accessibility, and quality of population-based and personal oral health services

Dental hygienists working within the public, private, or nonprofit sectors must have skills to assess community health problems and evaluate outcomes of community health solutions. Dental hygienists working in community settings generally participate in a variety of assessment and evaluation activities. Examples of some of these roles and potential activities are shown in Figure 3–1 (see page 44).

OVERVIEW OF EPIDEMIOLOGY: POPULATION-BASED STUDY OF HEALTH

Public health dental hygienists involved in assessment and evaluation should become well versed in the basic concepts of epidemiology, which is a core science of community health. This section provides a basic overview of epidemiology. Table 3–1 (see page 45) provides the definitions of terms used in epidemiology and community health assessments.

Epidemiology is the study of the distribution and determinants of health-related states and events in specified populations and the application of this study to the control of health problems.[11] Epidemiologists consider the interactions and relationships among the multiple factors that influence health status and health problems.[12] Methods used in epidemiology and research are combined to focus on comparisons between groups or defined populations. Epidemiologists make comparisons by examining the occurrences of the health events, locations, times, and variations to assess the distribution and determinants of health events.[13] The principal factors analyzed in epidemiology are as follows:

◆ Distribution
◆ Population dynamics

- Oral health program director evaluates the attainment of goals, objectives, and performance measures set out in the oral health improvement plan for the state.

- Oral health policy analyst determines the number and geographic distribution of dentists statewide who participate in the Medicaid and state Children's Health Insurance Program (S-CHIP) program and provide oral health care to young children under five years of age.

- Oral health program administrator with a city health department assesses the oral health assets, needs, and resources of a metropolitan area.

- Oral health educator assesses the knowledge, attitudes, and opinions of a community about community water fluoridation to develop an oral health promotion campaign.

- Public health dental hygienist from a county health department assesses dental sealants in third-grade children in schools throughout the county.

- Oral health program manager evaluates the quality and outcomes of clinical preventive services in a school-based oral health program.

- Oral health service provider monitors oral health indicators in the neighborhood surrounding a community health center.

- Private practice dental hygienist, appointed to a state oral health advisory committee, evaluates the oral health indicators in the state and the annual performance of the state oral health program.

Figure 3–1. Examples of roles of public health dental hygienists in assessment.

- ◆ Occurrences
- ◆ Affected population
- ◆ Place characteristics
- ◆ Time
- ◆ Determinants

Epidemiology is based on a multifactorial perspective, with consideration given to the interacting relationships among host factors, agent factors, and environmental factors.[12, 14]

Host Factors

The host may be a person, an animal, or plant. **Host factors** relate primarily to susceptibility and resistance to disease through biologic immunity, instruction and knowledge, behavior modification, screening,

Table 3–1
Common Terms Used in Epidemiology

Term	Definition
Acute	Referring to a health effect, brief exposure of high intensity
Chronic	Referring to a health-related state, lasting a long time
Cohort study	The method of epidemiologic study in which subsets of a defined population can be identified and observed for a sufficient number of person-years to generate reliable incidence or mortality rates in the population subsets; usually a large population, study for a prolonged period (years), or both (Synonym: concurrent, follow-up, incidence, longitudinal, prospective study)
Cross-sectional study	A study that examines the relationship between diseases (or other health-related characteristics) and other variables of interest as they exist in a defined population at one particular time
Dichotomous scale	A measurement scale that arranges items into either of two mutually exclusive categories
Endemic disease	The constant presence of a disease or infectious agent within a given geographic area or population group
Epidemic	From Greek *epi* (upon), *demos* (people); occurrence in a community or region of cases of an illness, specific health-related behavior, or other health-related events clearly in excess of normal expectancy
Eradication (of disease)	Termination of all transmission of infection by extermination of the infectious agent through surveillance and containment
Etiology	Literally, the science of causes, causality; in common usage, cause
Incidence	(Synonym: incident number); the number of instances of illness commencing, or of persons falling ill, during a given period in a specified population; more generally, the number of new events (e.g., new cases of a disease in a defined population) within a specified period of time
Index	In epidemiology and related sciences, usually referring to a rating scale or a set of numbers derived from a series of observations of specified variables (e.g., health status index, scoring systems for severity or stage of cancer, heart murmurs, mental retardation)
Monitoring	Performance and analysis of routine measurements aimed at detecting changes in the environment or health status of populations; may imply intervention in the light of observed measurements

Table continued on following page

	Table 3–1
	Common Terms Used in Epidemiology *Continued*
Term	**Definition**
Morbidity	Any departure, subjective or objective, from a state of physiologic or psychologic well-being; in this sense, *sickness, illness,* and *morbid condition* are similarly defined and synonymous
Mortality	Related to death
Multifactorial etiology	Referring to the concept that a given disease or other outcome may have more than one cause; a combination of causes or alternative combinations of causes may be required to produce the effect
Occurrence	In epidemiology, a general term describing the frequency of a disease or other attribute or event in a population without distinguishing between incidence and prevalence
Pandemic	An epidemic occurring over a very wide area and usually affecting a large proportion of the population
Prevalence	Number of instances of a given disease or other condition in a given population at a designated time; when used without qualification, term usually refers to the situation at a specified point in time (point prevalence)
Prospective	A research design used that looks forward
Retrospective	A research design that uses a review of past events
Sensitivity	(of a screening test); proportion of truly diseased persons as identified by the screening test; is the measure of the probability of a correct diagnosis or the probability that any given case will be identified by the test (synonym: true-positive rate)
Specificity	Proportion of truly nondiseased persons identified by the screening test; a measure of the probability of correctly identifying a nondiseased person with a screening test (synonym: true-negative rate)
Surveillance	Ongoing scrutiny, generally using methods distinguished by their practicability, uniformity, and rapidity rather than by complete accuracy; main purpose is to detect changes in trend or distribution in order to initiate investigative or control measures
Trend	A long-term movement in an ordered series (e.g., a time series); an essential feature is that the movement, while possibly irregular in the short term, shows movement consistently in the same direction over a long term

Adapted from Last JM (ed): A Dictionary of Epidemiology, 3rd ed. New York, Oxford University Press, 1995.

and personal power. Age, gender, socioeconomic status, race, ethnicity, culture, genetic endowment, behavior, physiologic and nutritional state, previous exposure, and other factors influence susceptibility and resistance.

Agent Factors

Agent factors are the biologic or mechanical means of causing disease, illness, injury, or disability, such as microbial, parasitic, viral, or bacterial pathogens or vectors; physical or mechanical irritants; chemicals; drugs; trauma; automobiles; and radiation. Biology, marketing, engineering, regulations, and legislation can influence agent factors.

Environmental Factors

Environmental factors include physical, sociocultural, sociopolitical, and economic components. The media, greed, beliefs, occupation, food sources, geography, climate, housing, social roles, technology, and other factors can influence the environmental conditions.

The "epidemiologic triangle" depicts disease as the outcome of the interactions among host, agent, and environmental factors.[12] For example, the development and progression of dental caries is attributed to multiple factors.[15, 16] Figure 3–2 (see page 48) portrays the epidemiologic triangle, with dental caries shown as a multifactorial disease influenced by host, agent, and environmental factors.

Uses of Epidemiology

Health represents a general balance among host, agent, and environmental factors; health problems occur when the balance is threatened by changes in host, agent, or environment.[14] Prevention is concerned with maintaining or initiating a balance of these factors. Disease or health status depends on multiple factors, such as exposure to a specific agent, strength of the agent, susceptibility of the host, and environmental conditions.[12]

Epidemiology can be used to provide many pieces of data and information.[17] Epidemiologists in public health agencies are responsible for surveillance, investigation, analysis, and evaluation.[12, 14] The various uses of epidemiology are illustrated in Figure 3–3 (see page 49). The three classifications of epidemiologic studies are outlined in the Guiding Principles feature shown next. Figure 3–4 (see page 49) depicts some of the traditional characteristics of epidemiologic surveys.

Host factors
- Tooth enamel (crystal and mineral structure)
- Saliva (flow and composition)
- Immunity (response to pathogens)
- Host (individual beliefs, values, behaviors, habits, and customs)

Dental caries

Environmental factors
- Plaque (quantity and quality)
- Enzymes
- Minerals
- Bacterial substrate (fermentable carbohydrate in diet)
- Protective factors (fluoride in toothpaste, water, etc.)
- Socioeconomic factors
- Community norms and cultural factors
- Family and social support networks

Agent factors
- Bacterial biofilm
- Specific bacteria
  Streptococcus mutans
  Lactobacillus
- Other bacteria

Figure 3–2. Epidemiologic triangle: Dental caries is a multifactorial oral disease.

Guiding Principles

Classification of Studies in Epidemiology

- *Descriptive studies.* Involve description, documentation, analysis, and interpretation of data to evaluate a current event or situation

- *Analytical studies.* Identify the cause of diseases, disabilities, injuries, and deaths; determine that a causal relationship exists between a factor and a disease or condition

- *Experimental studies.* Are used when the etiologic mechanism of the disease is established and the investigator determines the effectiveness of altering factors; applying or withholding the supposed cause of a condition and observing the results

- Describe patterns among groups.
- Describe normal biological processes.
- Elucidate mechanisms of disease transmission.
- Describe the natural histories of acute and chronic diseases.
- Test hypotheses for prevention and control of diseases, injuries, disabilities, and deaths through special studies in populations.
- Evaluate services (e.g., community preventive services, population-based health promotion services, and clinical health services).
- Study nondisease health and social problems such as occurrences of intentional and unintentional injuries.
- Measure the distribution of health status, diseases, injuries, disabilities, births, and deaths in populations.
- Identify determinants (e.g., protective and risk factors) for death or acquiring diseases, injuries, and disabilities.
- Evaluate interventions and strategies to prevent and control diseases, disabilities, injuries, and deaths.
- Predict trends of diseases, disabilities, injuries, and deaths.
- Identify health assets, gaps, needs, problems, resources, solutions, and partnerships within the context of a community assessment.

Figure 3–3. Uses of epidemiology.

▨ CHANGING PERSPECTIVES OF HEALTH

During the 20th century, major transformations took place in the concepts of health and the understanding of the determinants of diseases, disabilities, and injuries. Many historical developments contributed to these

- Naturally occurring sample of population group
- Fairly large sample sizes
- Cross-sectional surveys used usually (include one time period)
- Longitudinal surveys used occasionally
- Measures chosen for assessment establish a specific level of disease, disability, or injury in a selected population
- Measures chosen should be in general use to enable comparisons of findings for different population groups
- Data generated from epidemiologic surveys are used to establish underlying etiologic factors and to derive possible preventive methods that lead to the development of hypotheses to be tested by controlled clinical trials

Figure 3–4. Traditional characteristics of epidemiologic surveys.

expanded visions and had a profound effect on the health of individuals and populations.[1, 2, 18] These developments contributed to changes in clinical health care and public health practice. Examples of these changes include:

- Changes in social conditions and mores, professional ethos, and social institutions
- Shifts in views of civil and human rights
- Recognition of environmental health and ecology
- Technologic changes influencing work, home, and life in communities (e.g., transportation, telecommunications, computing)
- Advancements in the biologic, physical, quantitative, social, and behavioral sciences

There was a broadening of the concepts of health promotion and disease prevention from an individual focus toward a human ecologic perspective.[17] Health promotion theory has moved toward a complex, holistic, interactive approach, with a systems orientation focused on healthy people living in healthy communities. Health promotion approaches have begun to embrace the principles of population health, social ecology, and community participation.[17, 20, 21] These transformations about the meanings of health, wellness, and quality of life as well as health problems within communities are continuing to evolve in the 21st century.

▨ CONCEPTUAL MODELS OF THE DETERMINANTS OF HEALTH

Many models describing the multiple factors that influence the broader dimensions of health in individuals and populations were developed in the second half of the 20th century. Multicausal perspectives of health and disease began to take precedence over monocausal models.[12] The epidemiologic triangle model waned as the emphasis on infectious diseases diminished in the later part of the century. The concept of a "web of causation" emerged as multifactorial perspectives grew, with attention focused on the various determinants of chronic diseases, disabilities, and injuries.

Hancock, proposing a comprehensive framework to better understand the **determinants of health,** described the **mandala of health,**[22] a model of the human ecosystem (Fig. 3–5). Its circular pattern symbolizes symmetry and wholeness. The confluent circles represent the multiple determinants of health. The center illustrates an individual whose total health and well-being are represented by the integration of mind, body, and spirit but not in isolation from other conditions. Within the global community of the biosphere, the individual is presented as only an element interdependent upon larger systems. These larger systems include the family and the community within society. All domains

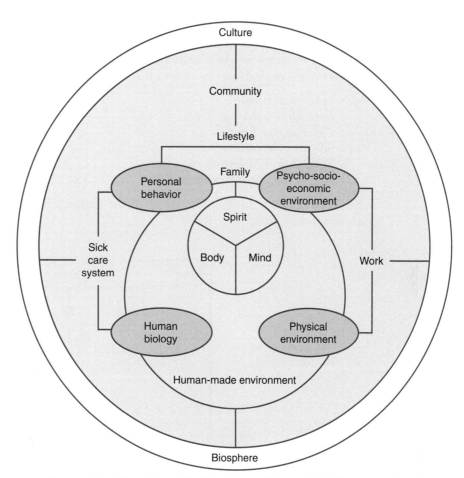

Figure 3–5. Mandala of health. (From Hancock T: The mandala of health: A model of the human ecosystem. Fam Commun Health 8:1, 1985.)

depicted in the model are surrounded and affected by ubiquitous cultural influences.

Also incorporated into the model are four groups of factors that influence the health of individuals, families, and communities:

* The psychosocioeconomic environment
* The physical environment
* Human biology
* Personal behavior

In the United States, a multidimensional perspective of health has shaped the development of the national health goals and objectives for *Healthy People 2010*. The decade-long strategy is based on a conceptual framework, the **systematic approach to health improvement.** This framework is grounded in the Force Field Model (see Fig. 3–6).[23] The Systematic Approach to Health Improvement framework describes the interrelated determinants of health. It includes the goals and objectives necessary to improve health. The determinants of health, according to this model, are classified as:

- ◆ Individual biology
- ◆ Individual behavior
- ◆ Physical environment
- ◆ Social environment
- ◆ Policies and interventions
- ◆ Access to quality health care

See Chapter 4 for further discussion of the national health objectives and *Healthy People 2010*.

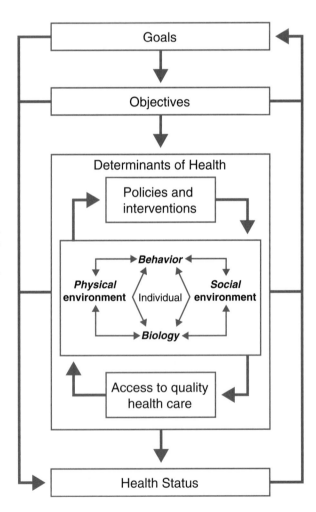

Figure 3–6. Conceptual framework from *Healthy People 2010* for a systematic approach to health improvement. (From U.S. Department of Health and Human Services, 2000.)

▨ DETERMINANTS OF HEALTH IN INDIVIDUALS AND POPULATIONS

The determinants of health have a profound effect on the health status of individuals, families, communities, nations, and thus the world.[6, 23, 24] The determinants of health are the factors that interact to create circumstances and produce specific health conditions; they can be classified as[1]:

- ◆ Physical (environmental)
- ◆ Biologic
- ◆ Behavioral
- ◆ Social
- ◆ Cultural
- ◆ Spiritual

These determinants may also be classified as follows[14]:

1. *Inherited* determinants are factors that are inborn or genetically determined.
2. *Acquired* determinants, which influence health and are obtained after birth and throughout life, include multiple factors such as infections, trauma, cultural characteristics, and spiritual values.

Many determinants of health influence the health of individuals and populations.[20-23, 25-30] Multiple determinants of oral health have been described in the literature.[16, 31] The boundaries between the specific categories of determinants are indistinct because they interact and influence each other continuously.[1, 14] During different stages of human development, the multiple determinants act synergistically, rather than separately, to affect health. No single determinant of health is the most important because multiple factors work in combination. Thus, causation is often described as multifactorial; that is, multiple factors determine health conditions, including diseases, disabilities, and injuries among individuals living in communities.

Several factors[14, 23, 33] are generally recognized as broader determinants of health (e.g., employment; education; environment; income; shelter; food; social justice and equity; family, friends, and social supports; peace and safety; culture and race relations).[22, 24, 32, 33] Other factors (e.g., language, learning, meaningful work, literature, recreation, self-esteem, personal control) are considered contributors to well-being.

A contemporary movement in public health called "Healthy Cities/ Healthy Communities" has accepted a broader multidimensional perspective of health.[19] The World Health Organization has promoted this concept, which focuses on the root determinants of health.[19, 15, 31, 34] Nations and communities around the world have adopted community health approaches based on this perspective.[19, 35] Healthy Communities groups ascribe to the following principles.

Guiding Principles

Healthy Communities: Perspective of Health[19]

* Broad definition of health

* Broad definition of community

* Shared vision from community values

* Quality of life addressed for everyone

* Diverse citizen participation and widespread community ownership

* "Systems change" emphasized

* Capacity built with the use of local assets and resources

* Progress and outcomes benchmarked and measured

The next topic is an overview of assessment as a key component within a comprehensive process that communities can adopt to improve health.

▣ THE PLANNING CYCLE

The **planning cycle** is a model commonly used in public health practice; it provides a basic flow chart of steps in a process to (1) **assess**, (2) **plan**, (3) **implement**, and (4) **evaluate**. Figure 3–7 shows a basic planning cycle. The planning cycle is continuous[2]; each stage can be further subdivided into detailed steps for a long-term health improvement process in the

Figure 3–7. Planning cycle.

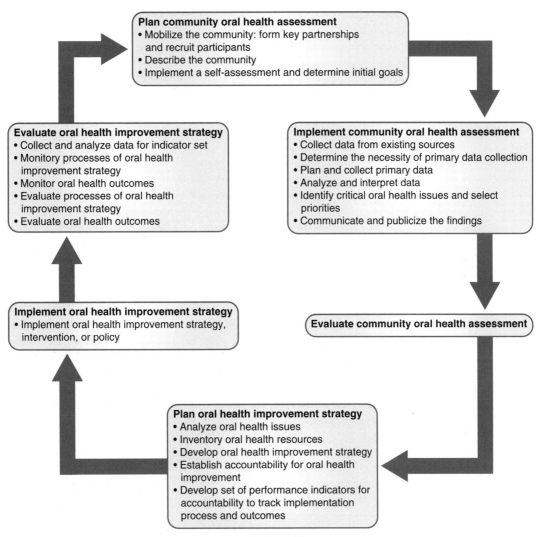

Plan community oral health assessment
- Mobilize the community: form key partnerships and recruit participants
- Describe the community
- Implement a self-assessment and determine initial goals

Evaluate oral health improvement strategy
- Collect and analyze data for indicator set
- Monitory processes of oral health improvement strategy
- Monitor oral health outcomes
- Evaluate processes of oral health improvement strategy
- Evaluate oral health outcomes

Implement community oral health assessment
- Collect data from existing sources
- Determine the necessity of primary data collection
- Plan and collect primary data
- Analyze and interpret data
- Identify critical oral health issues and select priorities
- Communicate and publicize the findings

Implement oral health improvement strategy
- Implement oral health improvement strategy, intervention, or policy

Evaluate community oral health assessment

Plan oral health improvement strategy
- Analyze oral health issues
- Inventory oral health resources
- Develop oral health improvement strategy
- Establish accountability for oral health improvement
- Develop set of performance indicators for accountability to track implementation process and outcomes

Figure 3–8. Community oral health improvement process.

community. The Community Health Improvement Process has been described as a comprehensive approach for communities to achieve sustained improvements in community health.[23]

Embedded into the basic planning cycle is a framework for a **community oral health improvement process** (see Fig. 3–8). Because of dynamics in community health, it is important to understand the necessity of flexibility in public health plans. If new circumstances arise, activities outlined initially in a plan may not be followed as sequentially ordered and work would need to be adjusted. However, it is important to include all of the steps for a community oral health improvement process.

Following such a planning cycle allows a systematic approach of assessing different factors, considering options for action, planning and implementing policies or programs, and evaluating their outcomes. This process can allow for coordinated community efforts in assessment, planning, implementation, and evaluation. When these efforts are institutionalized over time into the community fabric, long-term oral health benefits are likely to be achieved by the community.

⊠ ASSESSMENT OF ORAL HEALTH IN COMMUNITIES

This section reviews community oral health assessment, one component of a community oral health improvement process. It describes the steps undertaken and the indicators that can be included in an assessment.

A **community oral health assessment** is a multifaceted process that is community-oriented and community-directed. It focuses on population health, and it can concentrate on the entire population or a specific segment of the population in a community.

An oral health assessment considers assets, gaps, needs, problems, resources, solutions, and partnerships within the context of the community. Its purpose is to identify factors that affect oral health of a population and to determine the availability of resources and interventions that affect these factors. Communities are better served and improved outcomes are more sustainable when assets-oriented assessment methods are used, in contrast to deficiency-based approaches that focus on needs and problems. By engaging and fostering the community in a community-building process, one can gain insight about the specific factors in the community that influence health. Through a participatory framework for action and capacity development, a better understanding of opportunities for health enhancements can emerge over time.

With information gleaned from a broad-based assessment process, a community can begin to answer these questions about oral health:

- ◆ What community strengths, assets, and resources influence oral health in the community?
- ◆ What capacities, resources, and interventions are available within the community to promote oral health?
- ◆ What are the oral health problems, concerns, and obstacles faced by the community?
- ◆ What factors contribute to these community oral health gaps and needs?
- ◆ What are the potential solutions? What partnerships in the community can support strategies to ensure future oral health improvements?

Answers to these questions assist in final determination of critical oral health issues and priorities.

Assessment is the first, and an essential, step in the development of a community oral health improvement plan. The findings from the assessment can lead to the formation of oral health goals, objectives, plans, policies, interventions, and programs to solve oral health problems. Oral health programs best serve communities and address community oral health problems when priorities and actions are determined by current information and are grounded in evidence-based public health practices and contemporary principles.

Various community health assessment models have been used by communities. Many ways exist to collect information that can be used to evaluate the determinants of health for a population and a community. Numerous resources are available to describe methods and to offer guidance for community health assessments. Use of these resources can assist in a methodical approach to the assessment process in communities (see References and Internet Web sites at the end of this chapter).

One resource, developed by the Association of State and Territorial Dental Directors (ASTDD), is the ASTDD Seven-Step Model. This publication and videotape package provides a step-by-step guide for planning, implementing, and evaluating an oral health assessment.[10] The comprehensive guidebook outlines the main steps of a systematic and effective oral health assessment and reviews a broad array of alternatives that can be adapted for an oral health assessment.

No single formula exists for conducting a community oral health assessment. However, the ASTDD package outlines a useful model. An assessment should be developed on the basis of the specific aims as well as available resources, special circumstances, and expertise in the community. The essential components should be included in all community oral health assessments (Fig. 3–9) (see page 58). The essential elements are reviewed in more detail in the following section.

Planning a Community Oral Health Assessment

The first step in any assessment process is the planning stage. During this stage, it is important to methodically consider the overall purpose, potential partners, resources, and alternatives for conducting a community oral health assessment.

Mobilizing the Community: Forming Key Partnerships and Recruiting Participants

Community involvement is crucial in identifying oral health concerns and actions to resolve oral health problems. Collaborative partnerships and community coalitions are prominent strategies for community health improvement.[4, 35, 36a, 36b] Mobilization of community partnerships to identify and solve oral health problems has been identified as a key public health service to improve oral health in communities.[4] Community action and community-building efforts that engage and empower

A. Plan community oral health assessment

1. Mobilize the community: form key partnerships and recruit participants
2. Describe the community
3. Implement a self-assessment and determine initial goals

B. Implement community oral health assessment

1. Collect data from existing sources
2. Determine the necessity of primary data collection
3. Plan and collect primary data
4. Analyze and interpret data
5. Identify critical oral health issues and select oral health priorities
6. Communicate and publicize the findings

C. Evaluate community oral health assessment

Figure 3–9. Essential elements of a community oral health assessment.

communities can have positive outcomes when they are sustained over time.[7, 35] Contemporary public health practices and principles encourage multisectorial collaboration and broad community engagement to improve health-related conditions, outcomes, and well-being of entire communities[4, 23, 24, 30]

At the beginning and throughout a community assessment process, it is essential to involve diverse partnering agencies, organizations, associations, and individuals to collaborate.[37] Looking to the public, private, and nonprofit sectors may offer opportunities for potential champions of the assessment mission and process. Partners can broaden the scope, approaches, and perspectives in the process as well as provide community input, data sources, resources, expertise, and sponsorship. Partners can also lend support to collaborative community efforts that develop from the assessment outcomes. This may include support for communication of the findings and promotion of the strategies identified by the assessment. Engaging the community in the assessment process is key to building support for community oral health improvements. Involvement and support of partnering organizations throughout the assessment process can have a positive influence on the attainment of mutual missions and goals.

Potential partners should include a cross-section of the community, such as technical staff, program managers, and leaders from business, media, religious, civic, philanthropic, community, and political realms.[27, 38, 39] Appendix C outlines potential partners that can be supportive in community-based efforts, including an assessment. The partners should consider a broad spectrum of the community, and involve a wide variety of representatives of health and social service groups, organizations, and associations, governmental agencies and programs, community organizations, education-related groups (schools, colleges, universities), advocacy organizations, nonprofit, charitable and services groups, business organizations, and retail outlets.[27, 37–39] The partners involved in an assessment may vary according to the overall focus of the assessment process.[37]

Mechanisms for community participation, input, and dialog must be incorporated throughout the assessment process.[38] It is imperative to a successful community oral health assessment that the community be mobilized and actively involved throughout the process.[7] Broad-based community partnerships should be engaged and participants enlisted to reflect the cultural, racial, ethnic, gender, economic, and linguistic diversities of the community.[37] Procedures should be in place to ensure opportunities for communication with and feedback to the community, sustaining support throughout the process, and evaluation of the assessment.

It is important to consider ways of identifying and recruiting partners in the development of an inclusive and empowering process. Resource materials can be helpful by offering innovative ideas about building effective collaborative partnerships and community coalitions.[35] Many of these resources discuss in-depth ways to initiate and sustain vitality of collaborative relationships. Specific factors and conditions that are conducive to effective collaborative partnerships should be supported and nurtured for measurable and lasting results (see References and Internet Web sites at the end of the chapter).

Describing the Community

An important task of the assessment is to provide a description of the community, which must be clearly defined.[13, 27] Communities are a collection of peoples, places, and systems that define how people and places interact.[7] The "Guiding Principles" (see page 60) can be used to provide an understanding and a description of a community.

Initially, the description can include a general overview of the community but not detailed statistics at this point. More comprehensive, detailed community data should be compiled during the data collection phase. This information should be incorporated into the **community profile**, a comprehensive description of the community.[13, 20, 27] Examples of information in a community profile are presented in Appendix D.

Guiding Principles

Factors to Use in Understanding and Describing a Community[7]

* People (socioeconomics and demographics, health status, risk profiles, cultural and ethnic characteristics)

* Location (geographic boundaries)

* Connectors (shared values, interests, motivating factors)

* Power relationships (communication patterns, social and political networks, formal and informal lines of authority and influence, stakeholder relationships, resource flows)

Implementing a Self-Assessment and Determining Initial Goals

During the initiation of an oral health assessment process, it is worthwhile to conduct a self-assessment.[10] At this step of self-reflection, it is useful to conduct an internal assessment to evaluate your organization and to consider its role. It is important to make an external assessment by exploring the missions and roles of other organizations in the community. Organizational capacity, power structures, strategic plans, commitment, and resources should be considered during this phase.

The next step is to determine the goals of the assessment. The goals should come from the self-assessment and through a group consensus process among the partnering organizations. Before embarking on an oral health assessment process, partners must understand why the community is conducting an assessment and what the community hopes to achieve from it. It is important to clarify the scope and size of the assessment. The objectives and activities undertaken to achieve the goals of the assessment must be refined continually as information is collected and in light of available resources.

Implementing a Community Oral Health Assessment

Collecting Data from Existing Sources

Data collection is the gathering of information that the community can use to make decisions and to set priorities. Different types, sources, and levels of information are needed for a comprehensive assessment.[44-47] For a community health assessment, it is vital to collect information and evaluate data related to the current status of assets, gaps, needs, problems, resources, solutions, and partnerships in the community.[45-47]

A standard element of an assessment is the compilation and synthesis of existing data and information from secondary sources.[10] After existing information is assessed, a decision should be made about the collection of new information from primary sources.

WHICH DATA SOURCES ARE AVAILABLE?

Multiple resources of information are widely available to the general public. The sources of data used in an oral health assessment should be diverse to ensure a broad portrayal of the factors influencing oral health in the community.[10, 16, 40–43] A variety of data resources should be tapped to compile and review information during the data collection process.[44–47] Government agencies and private and nonprofit organizations produce and compile excellent reports on the various determinants of health and oral health. Sources of local information include local reports, literature reviews, magazines, newspapers, newsletters, maps, and marketing data. It is also important to review previous assessments that have been conducted in the community. Table 3–2 (see page 62) outlines examples of various sources of information for community health assessments. Examples of government resources for health data are provided in Appendix D.

During data collection, it is important to systematically conduct a broad search of available information and to organize an inventory of this information. It is essential to carefully compile the information from secondary sources and to establish a system to record, process, and organize the data and information.

WHAT TYPES OF INFORMATION SHOULD BE INCLUDED?

Different types of information are necessary to ensure that a complete assessment accurately describes the factors influencing health in the community.[7, 12, 14, 44] Community health assessment efforts can accomplish the following[44]:

1. Evaluate determinants of health.
2. Assess needs and assets.
3. Quantify vulnerable population groups.
4. Measure preventable disease, injury, disability, and death.

Two main classes of data are used to describe a community and to characterize dimensions of health within the community:

1. **Quantitative data** refer to information that is objective and measurable. The data can be expressed in a quantity or amount (e.g., the percentage of children with dental sealants or the percentage of young children with dental caries.[6, 10, 16, 40] These data numerically represent the size of a problem and determine its statistical significance. Data may include demographic information and vital statistics, such as numbers of births or deaths, incidence or prevalence rates of disease, number of schools in a county, and employment statistics.

2. **Qualitative data** refer to information that reflects the quality or nature of things that cannot be numerically measured or analyzed.[42] Qualitative data add meaning to the numbers and help to answer the question of

Table 3–2 **Sources of Information**	
Potential Source	**Example**
Federal, state, and local government agencies (see Appendix D)	◆ Health department, human services, and social services department, aging, disabled, highway safety, police departments (documents, reports, surveys, statistics) ◆ Population surveys ◆ National, state, and local health surveys ◆ Surveillance system; reports and records ◆ Population-based registries ◆ Health agency records and reports of participants enrolled in programs ◆ Agency records and reports of health professionals, health professional shortage areas, and community health centers ◆ State or local child protection agency records ◆ Environmental agency records and reports
Private and public (community) health, health care (clinical or personal health care), social, and human service programs	◆ Hospitals, health plans (health insurance claims data), health care systems (health charts and dental records, pathology reports), professional associations, trade groups, community advisory committees, community collaborative groups and coalitions (community surveys), health and social service groups, organizations, societies, associations (documents, reports, surveys, statistics)
Philanthropic, nonprofit, and charitable organizations	◆ Religious organizations and groups, voluntary agencies; civic organizations; service and voluntary groups; community organizations, advocacy groups (documents, reports, surveys, and statistics, local information and referral service inventories)
Schools and colleges	◆ School districts; school boards; school campuses; colleges; universities (student statistics, school health reports, school entry records)
Businesses, employers, and business organizations	◆ Major employers or chambers of commerce; marketing data and survey data (e.g., Claritas, National Planning Data Corporation); economic statistics and financial records, corporate annual reports (e.g., sales of drugs, foods, tobacco)
Media	◆ Media sources (television, radio, Internet, newspapers, magazines, newsletters)

why a problem exists in a community. Data may include information gleaned from personal interviews, descriptions of traditions and the history of a community, and information gathered from participant observations or focus groups.[10, 16, 27, 41–43]

The types of data collected, as well as the selection of a data collection method and instrument used, depend on the aims of an assessment and the resources available for the assessment.[10, 13] Various data collection methods and instruments are indicated for specific types of assessments. Each method has advantages as well as limitations.[10, 42] Table 3–3 lists the diverse data collection methods, instruments, and applications used in community assessments.

A spectrum of health indicators can be used to profile the health of a community.[44] Data collected for a "snapshot" in a community health assessment can describe:

- Population characteristics
- Summary measures of health status in the community
- Leading causes of death
- Measures of birth and death
- Measures of disease, injury, and disability
- Vulnerable populations
- Environmental health
- Use of community preventive services and personal health services
- Protective factors and risk factors for disease, injury, disability, and death
- Access to public health (e.g., community preventive services), personal health care, and social service system in the community

A new national health assessment tool, the Leading Health Indicators, was unveiled along with *Healthy People 2010*, the health goals for the decade in the United States.[6] These first-ever Leading Health Indicators include 10 areas, based upon the *Healthy People 2010* objectives. These measures allow Americans to easily assess the overall health of the nation and their communities to make comparisons and improvements over time. The 10 Leading Health Indicators cover the following[6]:

- Physical activity
- Overweight and obesity
- Tobacco use
- Substance abuse
- Mental health
- Injury and violence
- Environmental quality
- Immunizations
- Responsible sexual behavior
- Access to personal health care

The Leading Health Indicators are supported by 21 specific measurable objectives that reflect the influence of behavioral and environmental factors

Text continued on page 68

Table 3–3
Summary of Data Collection Methods*

Method	Instrument	Cost and Time	Advantage
Document Study			
Review and evaluate existing documents or records describing past events or occurrences.	Information abstracted from archival sources (raw data, datasets of summary data, printed reports); qualitative or quantitative data from public legislative bodies, governmental officials and agencies, private businesses, professional and community organizations, nonprofit foundations	$–$$ 🕐–🕐🕐	Data often readily available
Observational Field Study			
Assessment of actual events, objects, or people in "natural" setting.	Assessors use checklist, evaluation forms, camera, tape recorder, rating scales, observation field notes. Qualitative approach with content or situational analysis	$$ 🕐🕐	First-hand information
Windshield or Walking Tour			
Within community-designated boundaries, observers and recorders drive or walk in community areas at varying times of days and days of week to assess community activities, interactions and events through observation, informal conversations, and interactions with community members	Observers and recorders document community characteristics and record information using observational guide, checklist, survey tools, notes, photos, audiotapes, videotapes; qualitative approach with content or situational analysis; results summarized and displayed through written narratives, tables, diagrams, slide and video shows, maps, collages	$–$$ 🕐–🕐🕐	First-hand information

		Cost and	
Method	**Instrument**	**Time**	**Advantage**
Mailed Survey			
Assessment conducted by mail; adaptations include questionnaire sent home with children from school, Fax survey, magazine or newsletter survey, or electronic survey (using networked computers or Internet)	Self-administered standardized, structured questionnaire with closed-ended and open-ended questions completed by respondent; quantitative approach with statistical analysis of responses	$$ 🕐🕐	Data can be collected from a large sample
Telephone Interview			
Survey interview conducted by telephone	Interviewer reads structured interview schedule (standardized, questionnaire) with closed-ended and open-ended questions to respondent; quantitative approach with statistical analysis of responses	$$ 🕐🕐	Data can be collected from a large sample
Person-to-Person Interview			
Survey interview conducted face to face between a respondent and an interviewer	Structured interview schedule (standardized, questionnaire) with closed-ended and open-ended questions read to respondent by an interviewer; quantitative approach with statistical analysis of responses	$$–$$$ 🕐🕐– 🕐🕐🕐	Face-to-face communication allows for more in-depth information
In-depth Personal Interview			
Survey conducted face to face to learn about life history, events, and experiences	Interviewer uses open-ended, flexible, unstructured nondirective questions; transcriptions of tape recordings used for thematic analysis of content	$$–$$$ 🕐🕐– 🕐🕐🕐	Smaller sample with expanded perspectives
Screening Survey			
Rapid assessment using screening procedures	Standardized written criteria and measurements, measuring instruments, and protocols; cursory inspection provides crude estimates; quantitative approach with statistical analysis of results	$$ 🕐🕐	Practical and uniform information in a short time period

Table 3–3
Summary of Data Collection Methods* *Continued*

Table continued on following page

Table 3–3
Summary of Data Collection Methods* *Continued*

Method	Instrument	Cost and Time	Advantage
Epidemiologic Survey			
Extensive assessment using examination procedures, clinical samples, and clinical tests	Standardized written criteria and measurements, measuring instruments, and protocols; detailed planning of examination conditions, indices, criteria, sampling approach, personnel training, data collection, data management, and analysis; quantitative approach with statistical analysis of results	$$–$$$ 🕐🕐– 🕐🕐🕐	More detailed information
Asset Maps			
Geographic study and mapping that can identify patterns of community characteristics, physical assets, or settings of human activity and interactions	Input and display of data from existing sources or new data onto geographic map using simple materials (land use map and adhesives or pushpins) or detailed community planning and evaluation computer software (e.g., Geographic Information System [GIS] software) and other powerful tools for organizing location, distribution, and mapping of spatial data	$–$$–$$ 🕐–🕐🕐	Good overview and visualization of information
Inventories or Directories			
Documenting and cataloging of assets and capacities of individual community members or community resources, such as institutions, organizations, and associations	Identify, evaluate, and organize assets and capacities in a community and develop adequate mechanisms for linkages that can produce opportunities for action; such capacities may include assets owned or skills processed by individual community members; may also include sources of mutual aid, connections, and resources among institutions, organizations, and associations in a community	$–$$ 🕐–🕐🕐	Data often previously collected

	Table 3–3		
	Summary of Data Collection Methods* *Continued*		
Method	**Instrument**	**Cost and Time**	**Advantage**
Focus Group Guided group discussion provides information on a specific topic from a certain population group	Moderator leads guided group discussions among 5 to 12 individuals over ½ to 1½ hours by using a series of open-ended questions on a preestablished discussion guide; transcriptions from tape recordings and written field notes of discussions used for thematic analysis of content	$$–$$$ 🕐🕐– 🕐🕐🕐	Varied and ample information
Public Forum or Community Dialog Event Individuals or groups provide verbal input or feedback on specific issues	Moderator solicits, collects, and summarizes written comments or oral testimony; oral testimony recorded by tape recorder or court reporter to generate official record for analysis	$$ 🕐🕐–	First-hand and ample information
Community Visioning Process Groups of community stakeholders collectively develop shared vision of their community in the future	Through an interactive approach (retreat or workshop format), a skilled facilitator brings individuals together over one or more days and guides participants through vision process by posing questions and assisting participants to visualize the future community; small groups discuss visions and images; creation of document to reflect visions; follow-up meeting held to refine visions and to develop plan for incorporation of visions into community planning process	$$–$$$ 🕐🕐– 🕐🕐🕐	Broad with ample and varied input

Table continued on following page

| | | Cost and | |
Method	Instrument	Time	Advantage

Table 3–3
Summary of Data Collection Methods* *Continued*

Creative Assessment

| Community members document perceptions of community through creative means | Creative techniques and forums for expression (photography, film, theater, music, dance, murals, puppet shows, storytelling, drawings) used to convey wide range of perceptions of a community | $$–$$$ ☺☺– ☺☺☺ | Interesting and innovative |

* Consider assessment methods that can stimulate dialog, reflection, and action to improve community health.
  Key: $, Inexpensive; $$, moderate cost; $$$, expensive; ☻ , less time-consuming; ☻☻ , moderately time-consuming; ☻☻☻ , very time-consuming.

and community health interventions. These objectives can be assessed by states and communities to assess their current health status and to monitor changes over time. Examples of information for a community health assessment are presented in Appendix D.

Chapter 4 reviews specific measures that can be used in an assessment of oral health in a community and details the *Healthy People 2010* initiative.

Determining the Necessity of Primary Data Collection

A key step in the assessment process is determining the need for additional data and information.[10] This decision should be made on the basis of:

1. A reevaluation and possible refinement of the assessment goals.
2. An analysis of the findings from the existing data sources.
3. Available resources to support future assessment activities.

The partners determine and prioritize information needs and evaluate alternative methods of data collection. One option might be the integration of specific measures into ongoing surveys and assessments. Sometimes it may be necessary to collect original data.

During this phase, it is crucial to study the many alternative ways by which data can be collected for community health assessments. It is essential to consider both the advantages and disadvantages of the data collection options that are available to the group. After this analysis, the group strategically determines the final goals according to identified priorities and resources.

Planning and Collecting Primary Data

When it is necessary to collect original data, the partners develop a work plan that outlines the objectives, activities, roles, responsibilities, budget, and timetable.[10] Once the scope of the assessment is determined, methods can be selected and criteria defined in preparation for the primary data collection phase. Examples of tasks that should be considered for conducting primary data collection are listed in Appendix D.

Analyzing and Interpreting Data

Analysis and interpretation of data often require knowledge and experience, and this is where the backgrounds and experience of community members, representatives of partnering organizations, and professionals in the community are invaluable. Partners can call upon local community members to enlist their expertise and assistance in validating impressions and interpretations of the data examined for the assessment.

To analyze and interpret both primary and secondary data, numerous steps are necessary. The initial step is to synthesize the information and summarize the findings. Data collected must be analyzed to determine meaning and significance.[10] A critique of each data source is required to assess its trustworthiness. The partners must consider the limitations of the data and data sources by checking for potential errors or biases. It is important to consider the sampling technique, such as type of sample, sample size, participation of population segments, and generalization of findings to population groups based on the sample.

Because potential errors can be made in collecting, recording, and analyzing data, it is essential to review the data collection process to check that protocols have been followed to ensure standardization and to reduce the potential of bias or variation. The partners should evaluate that methods and techniques were in place to collect information consistently, record and compile information accurately, and analyze data completely and appropriately. Information should be reviewed carefully to consider the possibility of misinterpretation, errors in coding and groupings, erroneous instructions, or typographical errors.

When the data have been determined to be reasonably free of errors, they should be compared with other data. The partners ensure that the data being compared are alike as possible. Data of a community can be compared with those of surrounding communities, other counties, the region, the state, or the nation. It may be worthwhile to compare data with those of a baseline source, such as the *Healthy People 2010* objectives (see Chapter 4). Analysis of trends can be included by comparison of new data in one time period with data from previous years. This comparison may show changes in the community over a specific time period. Also, data showing changes among communities over time can be very useful for planning purposes.

The group determines whether there are opportunities to analyze existing data sets further. If existing data sets are available and additional analysis will generate new information, this alternative may result in more insight. In addition, the group might add or integrate the collection of new types of data into ongoing data collection efforts.

The group assesses the significance of the data collected; the term significance means that the information truly reflects a problem existing in a community. Studying the data for significance means that possible misleading findings are identified before conclusions are drawn from the findings. An abundance of data combining different data types allows for an easier determination of the significance of the findings.

Numerical calculations are made through statistical analysis for data collected by means of quantitative methods. A mathematical method is used to calculate relationships among quantitative variables to determine statistical significance. The calculations show whether the observed relationships among the variables happened by chance or not by chance (see Chapter 6 for an explanation of data analysis in research).

The relationships among data collected by qualitative methods are not calculated through statistical analysis. Data collected by qualitative methods are reviewed to identify common or unique themes from responses or observations. Using specific methods and professional experience, the partners assess the information contextually to answer the following questions:

- Does this information reflect a real relationship, or did it just happen by chance?
- Does this information indicate a pattern of themes in the population, or does it reflect a single individual's experience?

The partners consider the implications of the data by evaluating the meaning of the data within the context and expectations of the community. The findings can provide direction to future actions to build on community assets. With potential strategies indicated, this step may move the assessment phase toward the planning stage of a community oral health improvement process. At the same time, additional questions may arise that may direct the process toward the need for more information and supplementary assessment activities.

Identifying Critical Oral Health Issues and Selecting Priorities

In conjunction with the community, it is essential to identify critical oral health issues. During this stage, it is important to consider the identified assets, gaps, needs, problems, resources, solutions, and partnerships in the community. During the assessment process, community partners should evaluate the community's assets and resources to create a shared vision of change.[45] This encourages greater creativity when community partners begin to address problems and obstacles.

Community partners should be actively involved in all aspects of determining and prioritizing the critical issues. On the basis of all the evidence, it is crucial to analyze the situation and to determine the priority of oral health problems to be addressed in the future. Through a deliberative process, the community partners must reach a consensus about long-term and short-term solutions to address the identified oral health problems.

Key steps to determine and prioritize community oral health issues include the following:

1. Develop a prioritization process. Community input is vital in this process.
2. Ensure clear determination of oral health priorities in conjunction with the community.
3. Determine the community's capacity to address oral health priorities. Consider the assets and resources that were located during the assessment process. How can the wide array of community assets and resources be expanded and maximized to address the oral health issues?
4. Consider how amenable each oral health priority is to change. What realistic degree of change can the community achieve in a specific time period?
5. Assess the economic, social, and political issues that influence the community's ability to address the priority oral health issues. When formulating oral health improvement strategies to address public health priorities, be cognizant of economic, social, and political factors that can affect plans and strategies.
6. Identify community programs currently addressing oral health priorities that were identified through the assessment efforts. Consider expanding partnerships and building upon successful strategies. This may allow for more effective and efficient use of limited resources.

Communicating and Publicizing the Findings

It is essential to establish a plan to communicate and disseminate the findings. The partners present the findings from the data collection and analysis and share information about the overall assessment quest. These findings should be publicized and distributed widely to various community members using the diverse channels of communication available, such as public forums, news conferences, and publications. Components of a report can include a statement of the purpose, materials and methods used, results, a discussion, conclusions, a summary, and an abstract. An executive summary and a full report may be useful to communicate the findings.

The outcomes should be communicated in a straightforward manner. It is important to summarize the findings by highlighting key findings and by including the outcomes of the inventory of community assets and resources to emphasize the availability of resources as well as to note the limitations of existing resources in the community. It is helpful to illustrate the findings through charts, graphs, and tables. In addition, partners can provide the audience with a frame of reference to show how the community data compare with similar data from other local, state, or national figures. It is vital to explain the limitations of the data.

Chapter 7 describes contemporary strategies for promoting community oral health and communicating oral health findings.

Evaluating the Assessment Process

As with any process, it is important to incorporate evaluation. Throughout the oral health assessment process, the collaborating partners should, on a systematic basis, step back and evaluate the process.[10] Allowing time for evaluation along the way can provide opportunity to implement changes and to improve the process. Recording a critique of the assessment at the end of the process can allow a feedback loop in which lessons can be learned for future health assessments in the community.[10]

NEXT STEPS: DEVELOPING AND IMPLEMENTING AN IMPROVEMENT PLAN

With the published report of the assessment disseminated and the priorities identified, it is time to move to the next phase of the community oral health improvement process. At this stage, oral health improvement strategies can be developed to address the prioritized oral health issues outlined in the oral health assessment. Concrete goals, objectives, policies, and programs can be planned and implemented based on the findings, evidence, and priorities from the oral health assessment.

A community oral health assessment is virtually useless unless the information is used to develop and implement effective community oral health strategies. *Healthy People 2010* (see Chapter 4) can provide guidance in the development of an oral health improvement plan.

Summary

Assessment is a core public health function, and dental hygienists involved in public health practice must be proficient in the various aspects of oral health assessment. Assessment is an integral component of a community oral health improvement process. Information gained from a community assessment can be used to plan, implement, and evaluate oral health improvement strategies.

Community health assessment efforts are applied to evaluate assets, gaps, problems, resources, solutions, and partnerships in the community. This allows a community to assess the determinants of health, evaluate needs, quantify vulnerable population groups, and measure preventable disease, injury, disability, and death. A systematic approach is crucial to accomplish a comprehensive community oral health assessment. This chapter has reviewed the key elements necessary when a community undertakes an assessment. Data collection methods and instruments are varied, and their application depends on the overall aims of the assessment in the community.

The chapter has reviewed how epidemiology involves a multifactorial perspective to analyze the interacting relationships among host factors, agent factors, and environmental factors that contribute to health in populations. As the concepts of health broaden and the information age grows, it will be essential that dental public health professionals be skilled in working with communities to assess the determinants of oral health.

APPLYING YOUR KNOWLEDGE

1. Illustrate the determinants of oral health for the following groups and situations:
   a. Oral cancer among older adults in a county
   b. Early childhood caries among preschool children in a state
   c. Periodontal disease among disabled young adults in a region of a state
   d. Dental caries among adolescents in a city without fluoridated drinking water
   e. Adults without access to annual dental visits in a rural county
   f. Dental injuries among schoolchildren in a neighborhood
2. Group discussion: Read over the following situations and discuss your answers within small groups.

A: The social worker from the County Agency on Aging calls you to discuss the dental problems of the senior citizens attending local nutrition sites near your community health center. The state health department has recently distributed the State Oral Health Improvement Plan, which notes a high rate of oral cancer among older men and a low rate of dental attendance for older edentulous adults. How would you maximize these "windows of opportunity" to initiate a community oral health assessment? Whom would you contact? What steps would you take? Do you think these efforts could advance the development and implementation of a community oral health improvement plan?

B: At a local child care conference, a prominent speaker describes the high rate of early childhood caries among preschool children attending Head Start programs in the city. Also, during the conference, the new Director for the Supplemental Food Program for Women, Infants, and Children (WIC) from the local health department highlights the need to improve the nutrition, health, and dental education for families enrolled in WIC. After the conference, the Community Coalition for Healthy Children (CCHC) asks you to join as a representative of the local component of the American Dental Hygienists Association. How would you maximize this opportunity to focus on oral health and young children? Whom would you contact? What steps would you take to initiate a community oral health assessment? How might the CCHC evaluate the assets, gaps, needs, problems, resources, solutions, and partnerships within the context of your community? How might this assessment promote the development and implementation of a community oral health improvement plan?

Dental Hygiene Competencies

Reading the material in this chapter and participating in the activities of Applying Your Knowledge will contribute to the student's ability to demonstrate the following competencies:

Community Involvement
CM.1   Assess the oral health needs of the community and quality and availability of resources and services.
CM.6   Evaluate the outcomes of community-based programs, and plan for future activities.

Health Promotion and Disease Prevention
HP.4   Identify individual and population risk factors, and develop strategies that promote health-related quality of life.
HP.5   Evaluate factors that can be used to promote patient adherence to disease prevention and health maintenance strategies.

References
1. Scutchfield FD, Keck CW: Principles of Public Health Practice. Albany, NY: Delmar, 1997.
2. Turnock BJ: Public Health: What It Is and How It Works. Gaithersburg, Md, Aspen, 1997.
3. Institute of Medicine, Committee for the Study of the Future of Public Health: The Future of Public Health. Washington, DC, National Academy Press, 1988.
4. Public Health in America. Washington, DC, Public Health Functions Steering Committee, 1994.
5. The Public Health Workforce: An Agenda for the 21st Century—a report of the Public Health Functions Project. Washington, DC, U.S. Department of Health and Human Services, Public Health Service.
6. Healthy People 2010: Understanding and Improving Health (Conference ed, 2 vols). Washington, DC, U.S. Department of Health and Human Services, 2000.
7. Centers for Disease Control and Prevention: Principles of Community Engagement. Atlanta, Public Health Practice Program, 1997.

8. Centers for Disease Control and Prevention: Framework for program evaluation in public health. MMWR Morb Mortal Wkly Rep 48(RR11)1, 1999.
9. Association of State and Territorial Dental Directors: Essential State Dental Public Health Services to Promote Oral Health in the United States: Guidelines for State and Territorial Oral Health Programs, 1997.
10. Association of State and Territorial Dental Directors: Assessing Oral Health Needs: ASTDD Seven-Step Model. Arlington, Va, National Center for Education in Maternal and Child Health, 1997.
11. Last JM (ed): A Dictionary of Epidemiology, 3rd ed. New York, Oxford University Press, 1995.
12. Timmreck TC: An Introduction to Epidemiology, 2nd ed. Boston, Jones & Bartlett, 1998.
13. Abramson JH, Abramson ZH: Survey Methods in Community Medicine, 5th ed. New York, Churchill Livingstone, 1999.
14. Last JM: Public Health and Human Ecology, 2nd ed. Stamford, Conn, Appleton & Lange, 1998.
15. Nikiforuk G: Understanding Dental Caries: Etiology and Mechanisms. New York, Karger, 1985.
16. Cohen LK, Gift HC (eds): Disease Prevention and Oral Health Promotion: Socio-dental Sciences in Action. Copenhagen, Munksgaard, 1995.
17. Green LW, Ottoson JM: Community and Population Health, 8th ed. Boston, McGraw-Hill, 1999.
18. Starr P: The Social Transformation of American Medicine. New York, Basic Books, 1982.
19. Lee PR: Focus on healthy communities: Healthy communities—a young movement that can revolutionize public health. Public Health Rep 115:114, 2000.
20. Huff RM, Kline MV: Promoting Health in Multicultural Populations: A Handbook for Practitioners. Thousand Oaks, Calif, Sage Publications, 1999.
21. Airhihenbuwa CO: Health and Culture: Beyond the Western Paradigm. Thousand Oaks, Calif, Sage Publications, 1995.
22. Hancock T: The mandala of health: A model of the human ecosystem. Fam Commun Health 8:1, 1985.
23. Institute of Medicine: Improving Health in the Community. Washington, DC, National Academy Press, 1997.
24. Institute of Medicine: Healthy Communities: New Partnerships for the Future of Public Health. Washington, DC, National Academy Press, 1996.
25. Spector RE: Cultural Diversity in Health and Illness, 5th ed. Upper Saddle River, NJ, Prentice Hall, 2000.
26. Hahn RA: Anthropology in Public Health: Bridging Differences in Culture and Society. New York, Oxford University Press, 1999.
27. Aspen Reference Group: Community Health Education and Promotion: A Guide to Program Design and Evaluation. Gaithersburg, Md, Aspen, 1997.
28. Waxler-Morrison N, Anderson J, Richardson E: Cross-cultural Caring. Vancouver, BC, University of British Columbia Press, 1990.
29. Mechanic D: Medical Sociology, 2nd ed. New York, The Free Press, 1978.
30. Amick BC, Levine S, Tarlow AL, Walsh DC (eds): Society and Health. New York, Oxford University Press, 1995.
31. U.S. Department of Health and Human Services (DHHS): Oral Health in America: A Report of the Surgeon General. Rockville, Md, DHHS, National Institute of Dental and Craniofacial Research, National Institutes of Health, 2000.
32. Flynn BC: Healthy cities: Toward worldwide health promotion. Annu Rev Public Health 17:299, 1996.
33. Roseland M (ed): Eco-City Dimensions: Healthy Cities, Healthy Planet. Gabriola Island, BC, New Society Publishers, 1997.
34. Duhl L, Hancock T, Twiss JM: A dialogue on healthy communities: Past, present, and future. Natl Civic Rev 87:283, 1998.
35. Roussos ST, Fawcett SB: A review of collaborative partnerships as a strategy for improving community health. Annu Rev Public Health 21:369, 2000.
36a. Berkowitz W, Wolff T: The Spirit of the Coalition. Washington, DC, American Public Health Association, 1999.
36b. Kaye G, Wolff T: From the Ground Up (companion workbook to The Spirit of Coalition). Washington, DC, American Public Health Association, 1995.

37. Community Roots for Oral Health: Guidelines for Successful Coalitions. Olympia, Wash, Washington Department of Health, Community and Family Health, 2000.
38. Kretzmann JP, McKnight JL: Building Communities from the Inside Out. Chicago, ACTA Publications, 1993.
39. McKnight JL, Pandak CA: New Community Tools for Improving Child Health: A Pediatrician's Guide to Local Associations. National CATCH Meeting, American Academy of Pediatrics, Community Access to Child Health (CATCH) Program and Asset-Based Community Development Institute, Institute for Policy Research, Northwestern University, CATCH 2000, Elk Grove Village, Ill, April 15–16, 1999.
40. Weintraub JA, Douglass CW, Gillings DB: Biostats: Data Analysis for Dental Health Care Professionals. Chapel Hill, NC, CAVCO, 1984.
41. Blinkhorn AS: Qualitative research: Does it have a place in dental public health? J Public Health Dent 60:3, 2000.
42. Bailey KD: Methods of Social Research, 4th ed. New York, The Free Press, 1994.
43. Marshall C, Rossman GB: Designing Qualitative Research, 2nd ed. Thousand Oaks, Calif, Sage Publications, 1995.
44. Health Resources and Services Administration (HRSA), Community Health Status Indicators Project (CHSI): Community Health Status Report: Data Sources, Definitions, and Notes. Washington, DC, U.S. Department of Health and Human Services, 2000.
45. Sharpe PA, Greaney ML, Lee PR, Royce SW. Assets-oriented community assessment. Public Health Rep 115:114, 2000.
46. Minkler M: Community Organizing and Community Building for Health. New Brunswick, NJ: Rutgers University Press, 1998.
47. Anderson E, McFarlane J: Community as Partner: Theory and Practice in Nursing, 2nd ed. Philadelphia, JB Lippincott, 1996.

Assessment Resources

American Public Health Association
http://www.apha.org

Association of State and Territorial Dental
Directors
http://www.astdd.org

Association of State and Territorial Health
Officials (State Healthy People 2010 Tool
Library)
http://www.astho.org

Coalition for Healthier Cities and
Communities
http://www.healthycommunities.org

Community Toolbox
http://ctb.ukans.edu

International Healthy Cities Foundation
http://www.healthycities.org

National Association of County and City
Health Officials: Mobilizing for Action
through Planning and Partnerships
(MAPP); formerly Assessment Protocol for
Excellence in Public Health (APEXPH)
http://www.naccho.org

National Maternal and Child Oral Health
Resource Center
*http://www.ncemch.org/oralhealth/
default.html*

Public Health Foundation
http://www.phf.org

U.S. Department of Health and Human
Services, *Healthy People 2010*
http://www.health.gov/healthypeople

Health Resources and Services
Administration (HRSA), Community
Health Status Indicators (CHSI) Project
http:www.communityhealth.hrsa.gov

HRSA and Health Care Financing Administration (HCFA), Oral Health Initiative
(OHI)
http://www.hrsa.gov/oralhealth/index.htm

Centers for Disease Control and
Prevention (CDC), National Center for
Chronic Disease, Prevention and Health
Promotion (NCCDPHP) Planned
Approach to Community Health (PATCH)
http:www.cdc.gov/needphp

CDC, Public Health Practice Program
Office (PHPPO) National Public Health
Performance Standards Program
(NPHPSP)
http://www.phppo.cdc.gov

CDC and ASTDD National Oral Health
Surveillance Systems (NOHSS)
http://www.cdc.gov/nohss

Measuring Progress in Oral Health

Jane E.M. Steffensen, RDH, MPH, CHES, BS

OBJECTIVES

Upon completion of this chapter, the student will be able to:

- Discuss the health goals and health objectives of *Healthy People 2010*

- Describe the oral health objectives of *Healthy People 2010*

- Discuss the measures that can be used to assess oral health status and access to services in a community

- Compare and contrast the clinical and nonclinical measures used in oral health surveys

- Describe the current status and trends of oral health in the United States

- Discuss the factors that influence oral health in populations

- Identify oral health disparities among population groups

Key Terms

Healthy People 2010

Quality of Life

Disparities

Index

Decayed, missing, and filled teeth (DMFT)

Decayed, missing, and filled surfaces (DMFS)

Association of State and Territorial Dental Directors (ASTDD) Basic Screening Survey

National Health and Nutrition Examination Survey (NHANES)

Community Periodontal Index (CPI)

National Health Interview Survey (NHIS)

Behavioral Risk Factor Surveillance Survey (BRFSS)

Status

Trend

Opening Statement

The Burden of Oral Diseases in the United States[1]

- ◆ *Of young children 2 to 4 years of age, 18% have already experienced dental caries.*

- ◆ *More than half (52%) of 8-year-old children and 78% of 17-year-old adolescents are affected by dental caries.*

- ◆ *Dental caries continues to burden adults, with 99% of seniors (65 years of age and older) with dental caries experience.*

- ◆ *More than 100 million persons in the United States do not have access to optimally fluoridated drinking water.*

- ◆ *Only 18% of children (9 to 11 years of age) have received dental sealants.*

- ◆ *Of adults (35 to 44 years of age), 22% have destructive periodontal disease.*

- ◆ *Of senior adults, 44% no longer have their natural teeth because of dental caries or periodontal disease.*

- ◆ *More than 30,000 Americans are found to have oral and pharyngeal cancer, and approximately 7800 people die of these cancers each year.*

- ◆ *Approximately 108 million Americans have no dental insurance.*

- ◆ *Of young children (2 to 4 years of age), 55% have not had a dental visit in the past year.*

- ◆ *More than two thirds (63%) of older adults (age 75 years and above) did not have an annual dental visit in the preceding year.*

- ◆ *Adults miss more than 164 million hours of work each year as a result of dental concerns.*

- ◆ *An estimated $60 billion was expected to be spent on dental services in the year 2000.*

▨ ORAL HEALTH ASSESSMENT: ESSENTIAL IN MONITORING COMMUNITY HEALTH

To ensure that a comprehensive profile of a community's health is depicted, oral health should be included in a community health assessment. When the health of a community is assessed, oral health is often found to be an important concern for both children and adults.[2] Oral and craniofacial diseases and conditions that can be assessed at the community level are listed as follows:

* Dental caries
* Periodontal diseases
* Edentulism (complete tooth loss)
* Oral and pharyngeal cancer
* Soft tissue lesions
* Craniofacial anomalies, including cleft lip and palate
* Malocclusion
* Orofacial injuries
* Temporomandibular dysfunction (TMD)

Multiple determinants influence oral health in populations.[3] The etiology and pathogenesis of diseases and disorders affecting craniofacial structures are multifactorial and complex. They involve the interplay among social, cultural, behavioral, environmental, and biological dimensions.[1] These factors contribute to the development and progression of oral diseases, conditions, and injuries.[1] In addition, various factors affect the access of population groups to community preventive services (e.g., community water fluoridation) and clinical dental services. These measures can prevent and control oral problems. In a community oral health assessment, it is worthwhile to evaluate key determinants that influence oral health status and access to services. The national health objectives of the document *Healthy People 2010* provide an important framework for the development of an oral health assessment at the state or local level.

▨ HEALTHY PEOPLE 2010: NATIONAL OBJECTIVES FOR IMPROVING HEALTH

Promoting health and preventing disease are important concepts in the United States. Therefore, the nation has developed a plan for the prevention of disease and the promotion of health, embodied in the publication called **Healthy People 2010**.[4] These national health objectives shape the health agenda in the United States and guide health improvements. The *Healthy People* initiative has been the nation's disease prevention and health promotion blueprint beginning in the 1980s. *Healthy People 2000 (HP 2000)* set measurable national targets to be achieved by the year 2000.[5] *Healthy People 2010 (HP 2010),* the third generation of national benchmarks, was launched in January 2000 and established national objectives to be reached by the year 2010.[4] The initiative originated in a 1979 report, by the U.S. Surgeon General, that established the precedent for setting national health objectives and monitoring progress over an interval of a decade.[6]

Healthy People 2010 was developed through an extensive goal-setting, consultation process that involved the Healthy People Consortium, a public-private alliance of more than 350 national membership organizations and 270 state, territorial, and tribal public health, mental health, substance abuse, and environmental agencies.[4] This national effort brought together national, state, and local agencies; nonprofit, voluntary, and professional organizations; businesses; communities; and individuals to focus on improvements in the health of all Americans.

The national objectives have served as a basis for the development of state and community plans to improve health. In the 1990s, most states and many localities used the *Healthy People 2000* framework to guide the development of health improvement plans and performance standards. It is expected that similar state and local initiatives will develop in the coming decade based on *Healthy People 2010*.

The *Healthy People 2010* framework is built on a systematic approach to health improvement[4] (see Chapter 3 and Fig. 3–6). The goals outlined in *Healthy People 2010* provide a general focus and direction and serve as a guide for the development of a set of objectives that will measure progress in health within a specified time period. The objectives focus on the determinants of health, which encompass the combined effects of individual and community physical and social environments. Also, the objectives consider policies and interventions used to promote health; prevent diseases, injuries, and disabilities; and ensure access to effective personal and public health services. The ultimate measure of success in any health improvement effort is the health status of the target population.

The *Healthy People 2010* initiative has a vision of healthy people in healthy communities. It aims to promote healthy behaviors, promote healthy and safe communities, improve systems for personal health and public health, and prevent diseases, injuries, disabilities, and disorders. *Healthy People 2010* provides a mechanism for monitoring and tracking health status, health risks, protective factors, and use of services.

Healthy People 2010 includes two overarching goals[4]:

1. To increase quality and years of healthy life by ensuring that people of all ages enjoy increased life expectancy and improved **quality of life**.
2. To eliminate **disparities** in health among different segments of the population, whether the disparities are related to age, gender, race and ethnicity, education level, income, disability, sexual orientation, or geographic location.

Ten Leading Health Indicators have been designated in *Healthy People 2010* and will be used as key measures for annual report cards on national health.[4] *Healthy People 2010* contains 467 objectives, grouped in 28 focus areas; each focus area has a specific overall goal (Fig. 4–1).

GOALS

Goal 1: Increase quality and years of healthy life.
To help individuals of all ages increase life expectancy and improve their quality of life.

Goal 2: Eliminate health disparities among different segments of the population.
These health disparities include differences that occur by age, gender, race, ethnicity, education, income, disability, geographic location, or sexual orientation.

FOCUS AREAS

Each focus area has a specific goal and multiple objectives:

1. Access to quality health services
2. Arthritis, osteoporosis, and chronic back conditions
3. Cancer
4. Chronic kidney disease
5. Diabetes
6. Disability and secondary conditions
7. Educational and community-based programs
8. Environmental health
9. Family planning
10. Food safety
11. Health communication
12. Heart disease and stroke
13. Human immunodeficiency virus infection
14. Immunization and infectious diseases
15. Injury and violence prevention
16. Maternal, infant, and child health
17. Medical product safety
18. Mental health and mental disorders
19. Nutrition and overweight
20. Occupational safety and health
21. Oral health
22. Physical activity and fitness
23. Public health infrastructure
24. Respiratory diseases
25. Sexually transmitted diseases
26. Substance abuse
27. Tobacco use
28. Vision and hearing

Figure 4–1. *Healthy People 2010* summary. (Adapted from Healthy People 2010: Understanding and Improving Health [Conference ed., 2 vols.]. Washington, DC, U.S. Department of Health and Human Services, 2000.[4])

▣ HEALTHY PEOPLE 2010: NATIONAL ORAL HEALTH OBJECTIVES

The national oral health objectives have defined the nation's oral health agenda and served as a road map for national benchmarks. These objectives are based on the latest research and scientific evidence related to oral health. They combine current information with contemporary public health principles to benefit the largest number of people in the United States.

The oral health objectives form the foundation of decision making and may foster resource allocation. They help drive action at national, state, and local levels toward the achievement of common oral health improvement goals. States, territories, tribes, and localities can use the framework to guide health plans for oral health improvements. The oral health objectives can shape the development and implementation of policies, interventions, and programs tailored to specific population groups.

The oral health objectives identify significant opportunities to improve oral health for all Americans by providing a focus for efforts in the public, private, and nonprofit sectors. These objectives provide a framework for measuring oral health indicators and progress toward achievement of targets.

Oral health has been a specific focus area in *Healthy People 2000* and *Healthy People 2010*.[4, 5] Oral health is integrated into many of the focus areas of the other 27 chapters in the *Healthy People 2010* objectives for the nation. Three major issues related to oral health and included in other chapters are:

1. Increasing the minority oral health work force for dentists and dental hygienists.
2. Providing oral health examinations and needed dental care for patients with diabetes.
3. Reducing deaths from oral and pharyngeal cancer.

Table 4–1 outlines the key topics of the *Healthy People 2010* national oral health objectives.

A National Oral Health Surveillance System (NOHSS) has been developed based on a set of eight standardized oral health indicators from *Healthy People 2010* (see "Guiding Principles" on page 86).[7]

NOHSS is a collaborative effort between the Division of Oral Health of the Centers for Disease Control and Prevention (CDC) and The Association of State and Territorial Dental Directors (ASTDD). NOHSS is designed to help public health programs monitor the burden of oral disease, use of the oral health care delivery system, and status of community water fluoridation on both a state and a national level. NOHSS includes indicators of oral health, guidelines for oral conditions and oral health care, information on state dental programs, and links to other important sources of oral health information.

Text continued on page 86

	Table 4–1	
	Healthy People 2010: Oral Health Objectives	

Oral health goal: To prevent and control oral and craniofacial diseases, conditions, and injuries and improve access to related services

No.	Topic of Objective	Measure to Monitor Objective
3–6*	Deaths from oral and pharyngeal cancer	No. of oral cancer deaths per 100,000 population
21–1	Dental caries experience	% of persons with ≥1 dft or DMFT
21–2	Untreated dental decay	% of persons with ≥1 dt or DT
21–3	No permanent tooth loss	% of persons with 28 teeth, no teeth extracted
21–4	Complete tooth loss	% of persons with all teeth extracted, edentulous
21–5	Reduce periodontal disease Gingivitis Destructive periodontal disease	 % of persons with ≥1 bleeding site % of persons with ≥4 mm LOA in at least 1 site
21–6	Early detection of oral and pharyngeal cancer	% of individuals with oral and pharyngeal cancer diagnosed at earliest stage
21–7	Annual examinations for oral and pharyngeal cancer	% of individuals with recent oral and pharyngeal examination past year
21–8	Dental sealants	% of persons with ≥1 sealant on permanent molars
21–9	Community water fluoridation	% of people served by community water systems with optimal levels of fluoride
21–10	Use of oral health care system	% of individuals with annual dental visit
21–11	Use of oral health care system by residents in long-term care facilities	% of nursing home residents with dental service within last year
21–12	Dental services for low-income children	% of low-income children and adolescents with preventive dental service within last year
21–13	School-based health centers with oral health component	% of school-based health centers with an oral health component
21–14	Health centers with oral health component	% of local health departments and community-based health centers with oral health component
21–15	Referral for cleft lip or palate	% of states with system for recording and referring orofacial clefts

Table continued on following page

Table 4–1 *Healthy People* 2010: **Oral Health Objectives** (Continued)		
No.	**Topic of Objective**	**Measure to Monitor Objective**
21–16	State-based surveillance system	% of states with an oral health surveillance system
21–17	Tribal, state, and local dental programs	% of state, tribal, territorial, and local health agencies with an effective public dental health program (directed by a dental professional with public health training)

* Numbers refer to the chapter and objective as referenced in *Healthy People 2010.* For example, 21–1 is Chapter 21, Objective 1.
DT, decayed permanent teeth; DMFT, decayed, missing, and filled permanent teeth; dft, decayed and filled primary teeth; dt, decayed primary teeth; LOA, loss of attachment.
Adapted from Healthy People 2010: Understanding and Improving Health (Conference ed, 2 vols). Washington, DC, U.S. Department of Health and Human Services, 2000.[4]

Guiding Principles

◪ Oral Health Indicators

◪   ◆ Dental visits

◪   ◆ Teeth cleaning

◪   ◆ Complete tooth loss

◪   ◆ Fluoridation status

◪   ◆ Caries experience

◪   ◆ Untreated caries

◪   ◆ Dental sealants

◪   ◆ Cancer of the oral cavity and pharynx

▨ MEASURING ORAL HEALTH AND ITS DETERMINANTS IN POPULATIONS

During the 1990s, steps were taken in the United States at the national and state levels to formulate a systematic approach for oral health data collection and reporting. The focus of these collaborative efforts among organizations and agencies was to promote oral health assessment and monitoring that could be applied in a wide range of environments. These efforts also stressed the importance of oral health program evaluation in light of contemporary public health principles. An important aim of these efforts has been the dissemination of procedures for collecting comparable data to assess oral health. A long-term goal includes an approach for continuous monitoring of oral health at the community level and expansion of indicators in the oral health surveillance system.

Results of these endeavors included the development of standard ways to monitor the national oral health objectives, an oral health needs assessment model, and documentation of methods to measure community oral health.[4, 5, 8–13] Selection of a data collection method for a community oral health assessment should be based on:

1. Information of interest (e.g., types, of conditions and factors to be assessed).
2. Social and demographics of the population and community.
3. Purpose of the assessment (e.g., how the data collected are to be used after the assessment).

Traditional nonclinical measures include face-to-face personal interviews and telephone interviews, although other nonclinical methods can be used to assess different factors influencing oral health.[11]

Clinical methods include basic screenings and epidemiologic examinations.[9, 11, 12, 14, 15]

Basic screenings involve the use of direct observation techniques established for visual detection and identification of gross dental and oral lesions in the oral cavity with a tongue blade, a dental mirror, and appropriate lighting.

Epidemiologic examinations entail the use of detailed visual-tactile assessment of the oral cavity with dental instruments and a light source in an oral health survey.

Basic screenings and epidemiologic examinations do not constitute a thorough clinical examination[9, 11]; they do not involve making a clinical diagnosis that would result in a treatment plan. Surveys are cross-sectional when they look at a population at a point in time. Surveys are descriptive, as they allow for oral health determinants to be ascertained and oral health status to be estimated for a defined population.

Common dental indices are used for clinical measures in oral health surveys. A dental **index** is an abbreviated measurement of the amount or condition of oral disease in a population. An index is based on a graduated numerical scale with defined upper and lower limits. It is an aid in data collection, allowing for comparisons among population groups that are classified by the same criteria and methods (see "General Principles" on page 88).

This chapter focuses on measurements of oral health that are used in population-based oral health surveys. The following text highlights common measures used to assess population oral health, specifies oral health indicators included in *Healthy People 2010*, and provides an overview of clinical and nonclinical data collection methods related to oral health assessment. The Dental, Oral, and Craniofacial Data Resource Center is compiling a catalog of oral health databases and an archive of oral health

Guiding Principles

 Attributes of a Good Index[16]

 ◆ Valid

 ◆ Reliable

 ◆ Clear, simple, and objective

 ◆ Sensitive to shifts in disease

 ◆ Acceptable to the participants involved

◆ Amenable to statistical analysis

assessment procedures. This resource center is funded by the National Institute for Dental and Craniofacial Research (NIDCR) of the National Institutes of Health (NIH) and the CDC's Division of Oral Health. Resources can be located on the NIDCR Web page.

Measures and methods used for assessment of individual patients in clinical settings or in clinical studies (including clinical trials) are not emphasized in this chapter. Other books review clinical evaluation techniques or clinical research methods.[17]

▦ TYPES OF MEASUREMENTS

Measurements of Dental Caries

Permanent Dentition

Dental caries (tooth decay) is an infectious disease that results in demineralization and, ultimately, cavitation of the tooth surface if the process is not controlled or if the tooth is not remineralized. This bacterial infection is influenced by a variety of factors in the host, agent, and environment. Unless dental caries is arrested early, the process is irreversible.

Dental caries can occur in primary or permanent teeth. General types of tooth decay include coronal (occurring on the crowns of teeth) and root surface (occurring on the roots of teeth). Coronal and root surface caries can be assessed by a systematic evaluation of teeth through epidemiologic examination or screening procedures. The status of **decayed, missing, and filled teeth (DMFT)** or **decayed, missing, and filled surfaces (DMFS)** is commonly recorded by a basic screening or oral epidemiologic examination.[9, 12, 14, 15]

The conventional DMF indices are used to count coronal caries of permanent teeth (DMFT) or surfaces (DMFS). Although the DMF Index has been used extensively in oral health surveys and has been a standard measurement in many countries, it is limited in its ability to measure thoroughly the characteristics of dental caries.[13, 15] As patterns of dental caries change, technology develops, and the goals of oral health surveys shift toward more situational analyses in communities, different approaches for the measurement of dental caries may emerge in the future.[9, 11]

For the DMF Index, each tooth space is scored as to whether it is sound or is diseased and whether there is evidence of treated or untreated clinical caries.[18, 19] In surveys of populations, the DMF Index is usually based on 28 permanent teeth. If ever diseased, the tooth must show one of three conditions:

1. Untreated, frank cavitation (decayed = D).
2. Evidence of restorative treatment resulting from caries (filled = F).
3. Evidence of a lost tooth due to caries (missing = M).

The DMF Index for an individual is the sum of either teeth (DMFT) or surfaces (DMFS) having these three conditions. The DMF Index is considered irreversible, as it indicates cumulative, lifetime caries experience and is used to measure past and present caries experience.

The **Association of State and Territorial Dental Directors (ASTDD)** has developed **Basic Screening Survey** methods through the Screening Training Project (STP). It assesses untreated dental caries and dental caries experience on a per-person basis.[9] Dichotomous measures (e.g., yes or no) are used during the screening of each individual to record the absence or presence of untreated dental caries as well as experience of dental caries (at least one decayed tooth, restored tooth, or missing tooth). Population measures are formulated to indicate the percentage of the population with untreated dental caries and dental caries experience. See Table 4–1 for a summary of the ways in which dental caries will be monitored for *Healthy People 2010*.

In oral health surveys, the terms *caries-free* and *caries experience* are commonly used to describe the status of population groups. When the DMFT score is equal to or more than 1, the person is considered to have experienced dental caries (at present, D; at some time in the past, M or F). When the DMDT equals 0, the person is considered to be caries-free. Population measures are used to indicate the percentage of the population with dental caries experience and, its complementary measurement, the percentage of the population that is caries-free. For example, a survey can show that 52% of children in the population have experienced dental caries and the other 48% are caries-free.

In the United States, oral health surveys typically have used a dichotomous scale for the diagnosis of coronal caries. Dental caries is scored by the presence or absence of a cavitated lesion based on established diagnostic criteria. According to the ASTDD Basic Screening Survey methods, untreated dental caries is detected and recorded by the screener on the basis of observation of the following two criteria[9]:

◆ A loss of at least 0.5 mm of tooth structure at the enamel surface
◆ Brown or dark brown discoloration of the walls of the cavity

Intraoral epidemiologic examinations can be used to assess the occurrence of root surface caries in oral health surveys.[19] Assessments of each tooth (and surface) present can be evaluated by scoring:

- Sound root
- Decayed root
- Filled root but with decay
- Filled root without decay
- Unexposed root (no gingival recession beyond the cementoenamel junction [CEJ])
- Bridge abutment/implant

The measurement of root surface caries in populations is generally based on the number of exposed root surfaces decayed or filled, with consideration given to the number of surfaces present in the mouth and at risk for dental caries.

Additional measurements of dental caries have been developed to reflect treatment needs and to provide a broader profile of the impact of dental caries in population groups.[14] A measure of selected restoration and tooth conditions was developed to supplement the DMF Index and to characterize the prevalence and severity of physical and biologic conditions that result from dental caries. The Restorations and Tooth Conditions Assessment (RTCA) was measured in the **Third National Health and Nutrition Examination Survey (NHANES III)**.[20] The RTCA was used to evaluate permanent teeth or tooth spaces of adults (18 to 74 years of age). For the RTCA, evaluations were recorded on the basis of the following criteria[20]:

- Soundness
- Defective intracoronal restorations, crowns, or bridges
- Gross loss of tooth structure associated with a restoration
- Pulpal involvement
- Retained roots

Scoring of teeth and tooth conditions for the RTCA is based on a hierarchical approach to measure severity by recording the worst condition.

Primary Dentition

The DMF Index can be modified for primary teeth in children.[18, 21] Indices commonly used for assessing the primary dentition include the df index or dmf index. The df index is the sum of decayed (d) and filled (f) primary tooth surfaces (dfs) or teeth (dft). It does not include missing teeth because of the difficulty in distinguishing primary tooth loss as a result of dental caries from those lost by natural exfoliation.

Note: Upper case letters (e.g., DMFT) signify *permanent* teeth; lower case letters (e.g., dft) signify *primary* teeth.

For use in children before the age of exfoliation (<5 years), the dmf index can indicate the number of teeth or surfaces with history of decay: d denotes decayed teeth, m denotes missing teeth resulting from caries, and f denotes teeth that had been previously filled.

For preschool-aged children the assessment of early childhood caries has been used in population-based surveys. To assess the "baby bottle tooth decay" pattern, an examiner evaluates a young child's six maxillary anterior teeth and determines whether one or more of the teeth are decayed, filled, or missing because of dental caries.[9] Missing front teeth for preschool children are most likely a result of caries or traumatic injury. Therefore, the cause of missing anterior teeth must be identified by questioning the parent or guardian, if present, during the screening or must include a question on the consent form. The ASTDD Basic Screening Survey methods outline assessment of early childhood caries for children under age 3 years.

Measurement of Dental Treatment Need

The World Health Organization (WHO) has established basic methods for oral health surveys in its "Pathfinder" approach.[15] WHO includes the assessment of treatment needs. During the epidemiologic examination, the examiner records a treatment need for each tooth separately and the treatment needs can be tabulated for population groups. Treatment categories include[15]:

- No treatment
- Preventive or caries-arresting care
- Sealant
- Restoration(s) (one or two or more surfaces)
- Crown for any reason
- Veneer or laminate
- Pulp care and restoration
- Indication for extraction
- Other treatment

For each person examined, the current status of a prosthesis and need for a prosthesis can be recorded by assessing the type of prosthesis needed and the arch in need.[14, 15] It is also common to assess need for dental care and referral.

The assessment of treatment needs may be problematic because it is difficult to standardize clinical judgments for the most appropriate treatment required on the basis of the treatment needs of the average person in the community. Findings of treatment needs can be useful for planning and monitoring purposes. They can be helpful in estimating personnel and service requirements, with demand levels for these services taken into consideration.

Summary assessments that record overall need for dental care (e.g., treatment urgency) are also used in oral health surveys. The ASTDD Basic

Screening Survey methods use the following three categories measured during a screening to assess need and referral for dental care[9]:

1. *None*—no obvious oral health problem; routine dental care (next regular checkup) recommended.
2. *Early*—observable oral health problem (dental caries without accompanying signs or symptoms, spontaneous bleeding of the gums, white or red soft tissue areas suggestive of a problem or ill-fitting denture); early dental care (within several weeks) recommended.
3. *Urgent*—signs or symptoms that include pain, infection, swelling, soft tissue ulceration of more than 2 weeks of duration (determined by questioning), emergency dental care (within 24 hours) recommended.

Measurement of Dental Sealants

Dental sealants are traditionally assessed in populations through a basic screening or epidemiologic examination procedure.[9, 22] Tooth surfaces and teeth can be evaluated for the presence or absence of dental sealants in the pits and fissures of erupted primary or permanent teeth. Sometimes oral health survey protocols limit measurements for dental sealants to selected tooth surfaces or teeth (e.g., permanent molars).[9] The screener can assess for the presence of dental sealants on a per-person basis using the ASTDD Basic Screening Survey methods.[9] This screening protocol focuses on the eight permanent molar teeth. During the screening, a dichotomous measure is used to assess for the presence or absence of dental sealants.

When a tooth is scored for treatment need in an oral health survey, the examiner can record the need for sealant or other preventive and caries-arresting care.[15] This measurement is included in the WHO Pathfinder methodology. This measure can be problematic, because criteria for dental sealant need and caries-arresting care have not been standardized for oral epidemiologic surveys.

See Table 4–1 for a summary of how dental sealants will be monitored for *Healthy People 2010*.

Measurement of Periodontal Disease

Gingivitis is characterized by localized inflammation, swelling, and bleeding of the soft tissues surrounding a tooth without loss of connective tissue or bone support. The condition results in swelling and bleeding of the gums. Gingivitis usually is reversible with proper daily oral hygiene, and its presence or absence serves as a crude measure of a person's self-care practices (e.g., toothbrushing).[23] Although not all occurrences of gingivitis progress to periodontal disease, all periodontal disease starts as gingivitis.[16] Destructive periodontal disease is manifested by the loss of the connective tissue and bone that support the teeth.[23] Destructive periodontal disease places a person at risk for eventual tooth loss unless appropriate treatment commences.

Contemporary indices to assess the health of periodontal tissues in population-based surveys reflect current theories of the pathogenesis of periodontal diseases. A disaggregated approach is taken to evaluate and record clinical signs of disease. Each measure is usually scored separately. Typical clinical signs that can be measured to assess periodontal status include[24]:

- Gingival bleeding
- Loss of supporting structure as a measure of past disease (recession or loss of periodontal attachment)
- Pocket formation
- Calculus as a contributing risk factor

For the oral epidemiologic examination procedures in NHANES III, explicit protocols and criteria were outlined for assessments of periodontal status.[28] In the epidemiologic examination, the examiner measured gingivitis using the gingival bleeding index by "walking" the probe inside the gingival sulcus to determine the number of sites of gingival bleeding. In addition, periodontal pocket depth on probing, calculus (supragingival or subgingival), and furcations were assessed in the epidemiologic examination. The measurements allowed for the calculation of recession and loss of attachment. The loss of clinical periodontal attachment is defined as the distance in millimeters between the CEJ and the bottom of the sulcus (e.g., periodontal depth minus the distance from the CEJ to the free gingival margin). The extent and severity of destructive periodontal disease are often measured by loss of periodontal attachment, pocket-probing depth, and furcation involvement.

See Table 4–1 for a summary of how periodontal disease will be monitored for *Healthy People 2010*.

The presence of at least one bleeding site has been used to define gingivitis in populations and is used to measure progress in *Healthy People 2010*. The occurrence of destructive periodontal disease is often measured by loss of periodontal attachment. The presence of one or more sites with loss of periodontal attachment of 4 mm or greater has been used to delineate destructive periodontal disease in a population. This measure has been used to monitor achievement of targets for the national oral health objectives, and it has allowed the monitoring of changes in destructive periodontal disease over time, distinguishing the status of one population from that of another.

A method of assessing periodontal health status, the **Community Periodontal Index (CPI)**, has been developed by WHO and is included in the WHO basic methods for oral health surveys.[15] It is a modification of the Community Periodontal Index of Treatment Needs (CPITN). The CPI allows for a rapid assessment of periodontal status of a population according to various grades of periodontal health.

The CPI divides the teeth into sextants for measurement. The severest measurement of the sextant is scored during an epidemiologic examination. The CPI provides a measurement of:

- Healthy gingiva
- Presence or absence of gingival bleeding
- Supragingival or subgingival calculus
- Periodontal pockets (*shallow*, 4 to 5 mm, and *deep*, 6 mm or more)

Loss of periodontal attachment is measured, and the highest score is recorded by sextant.

The treatment need codes for observed conditions were eliminated from the original CPITN because they did not reflect contemporary theories of periodontal diseases. The CPI calls for a specially designed lightweight probe with a 0.5-mm ball at its tip and bearing specific millimeter markings. In the United States, a modified version of the CPI, the Periodontal Screening Record (PSR) is used for screening in the clinical setting.[17]

Sometimes, to increase efficiency, to lower cost, and to decrease time spent on the epidemiologic examination, partial-mouth periodontal measurements are made to assess periodontal health. Historically, the Periodontal Disease Index (PDI) included specific index teeth to be measured, dubbed the "Ramfjord teeth."[16] The CPI identifies specific index teeth for different age groups.[15] Two quadrants (one maxillary and one mandibular) were randomly selected and specific tooth sites were measured for the periodontal examination in the NHANES III.[24] This method, used in NHANES III, allowed comparison with the periodontal findings from the National Survey of Oral Health in U.S. Employed Adults and Seniors, 1985–1986, conducted by the National Institute for Dental Research (NIDR) of the NIH.

Retention and Loss of Teeth

"No tooth loss" is equivalent to "tooth retention." "Complete tooth loss" reflects no remaining teeth regardless of the cause of the loss.[9, 25] Lack of any natural teeth is defined as edentulousness or edentulism. An individual with at least one natural tooth is considered dentate. Tooth retention and tooth loss can be measured in oral health surveys.[9, 15, 25]

The ASTTD Basic Screening Survey methods assess edentulousness on a per-person basis.[9] A dichotomous measure is used during the screening of each individual to record the absence of all natural teeth or the presence of all natural teeth.

In an epidemiologic examination, each tooth space can be assessed and scored to evaluate retention or loss of natural teeth.[15, 25] Data collected about the presence or absence of each tooth are used as indicators of tooth retention and tooth loss at the tooth level, arch level, or individual level for population studies.

Missing teeth can be assessed by tooth type and are scored by cause of loss (e.g., caries, periodontal disease, trauma, congenital absence, or orthodontia). However, determining the exact cause of tooth loss is difficult and can be problematic for a dental examiner. Assessment of tooth retention and loss can be made in the primary or permanent dentition. The missing primary tooth score should be used only in an age group in which normal exfoliation would not sufficiently explain tooth absence.

Furthermore, complete tooth loss can be tracked through interviews and constitutes the basis of the measures used for *Healthy People 2010*. Self-reported dentition status can be provided in a face-to-face interview or in a telephone interview. Two questions from the **National Health Interview Survey (NHIS)**, used in 1998, ask for edentulous status of each arch, and responses of "yes" to both questions determined complete tooth loss.[26] The questions are:

- Have you lost all of your upper natural (permanent) teeth? Yes No
- Have you lost all of your lower natural (permanent) teeth? Yes No

See Table 4–1 for a summary of the ways in which tooth loss will be monitored for *Healthy People 2010*.

Measurement of Oral and Pharyngeal Cancer

Data to measure the number of deaths due to cancer of the oral cavity or pharynx are obtained from death certificates collected through the National Vital Statistics System, within the National Center for Health Statistics (NCHS) of the CDC; such data are available at the state and local levels.[4, 13] This measure is based on the number of deaths per 100,000 people attributed to cancers classified in categories 140 to 149 of the 9th edition of the *International Classification of Diseases (ICD-9)*. Oral and pharyngeal cancers include cancers of the lip, tongue, buccal mucosa, floor of the mouth, and pharynx.

A second measure tracked is the proportion of oral and pharyngeal cancer lesions diagnosed at the earliest stage (e.g., stage 1, localized).[4] This measure is collected through state cancer registries and the Surveillance, Epidemiology, and End Results (SEER) of the National Cancer Institute (NCI) of the NIH. Specific factors related to population groups (e.g., age, gender, race, ethnicity) are often identified in assessments of oral and pharyngeal cancers in populations.

Another measure related to oral and oropharyngeal cancer is the receipt of an examination to detect oral and pharyngeal cancer. The National Health Interview Survey, used in 1998, assessed this action through self-reports.[26] The face-to-face interview included the following two questions:

- Have you ever had a test for oral cancer in which the doctor or dentist pulls on your tongue, sometimes with gauze wrapped around it, and feels under the tongue and inside the cheeks? Yes No
- When did you have your most recent oral cancer examination? Was it a year ago or less? More than 1 year but not more than 2 years? More than 2 years but not more than 3 years? More than 3 years but not more than 5 years? Over 5 years?

See Table 4–1 for a summary of how oral and pharyngeal cancers will be monitored for *Healthy People 2010*.

Measurement of Other Oral and Craniofacial Diseases, Conditions, and Injuries

Malocclusion and Craniofacial Anomalies

Malocclusion through evaluation of occlusal characteristics can be assessed during a population-based oral health survey. Some measurements focus on clinical measures of function, whereas other measurements are used to assess aesthetics.

The evaluation of occlusal traits was included in the epidemiologic examination protocol for persons aged 8 to 50 years for NHANES III.[27] It included measurements of incisor alignment, overjet, overbite, presence or absence of a posterior cross-bite, and presence or absence of a maxillary midline diastema. In addition, two questions were included in the face-to-face interview to ascertain the receipt of orthodontic treatment and age at initiation of orthodontic treatment.

WHO incorporates the *Dental Aesthetics Index* (DAI) in its epidemiologic examination protocol for a basic oral health survey.[15] The DAI considers an individual's social and psychological well-being as the main benefit of orthodontic treatment. It includes objective measurements of aesthetic acceptability according to social norms.[28] Clinical assessments of missing incisors, canines, or premolars are recorded along with the following evaluations:

- Crowding and spacing in the incisal segments of both arches
- Diastema
- Largest anterior maxillary and mandibular irregularities (rotations or displacements from normal alignment)
- Anterior maxillary and mandibular overjet
- Vertical anterior open bite
- Anteroposterior molar relation

In the United States, craniofacial anomalies (including cleft lip and palate) are usually expressed as a proportion or rate based on recordings of congenital anomalies in birth certificates.[29] Recordings of craniofacial anomalies and oral clefts on birth certificates may not be universal.

Orofacial Injuries

Tooth trauma can be assessed under oral epidemiologic examination procedures to evaluate clinical evidence of tooth injury and treatment received for the injury.[30] The NIDR Trauma Index was used in NHANES III among persons 6 to 50 years of age to assess, retrospectively, the outcomes of injuries to anterior teeth. The index was developed at the NIDR. The index tracks the status of the tooth, from sound (no evidence of trauma) through a missing tooth due to trauma, and reflects selected sequelae of trauma.[30]

The classification scheme measures seven levels of tooth trauma and is applied to each of the incisor teeth or tooth spaces. A history of trauma is obtained by questioning individuals in the sample, and assessments are recorded for the eight permanent incisors in children and adults.

Orofacial Pain and Temporomandibular Dysfunction

A temporomandibular joint assessment is included in the WHO basic oral health survey guide.[15] The guide suggests evaluation of signs such as the occurrence of clicking, tenderness on palpation, and reduced jaw mobility on opening greater than 30 mm during an epidemiologic examination. Brief interview questions are added to ascertain symptoms and include self-report of clicking, pain, or difficulties in opening or closing the jaw once or more within a week.

Dental Fluorosis

Dean's Fluorosis Index is the conventional index used to assess for dental fluorosis.[15] This index is one of the most universally accepted classifications for dental fluorosis. Each tooth present in an individual's mouth is rated according to these classifications: normal, questionable, very mild, mild, moderate, and severe. The classifications are based on specific criteria describing the enamel. The individual's fluorosis score is based on the severest form of fluorosis recorded for two or more teeth.

Dean's Fluorosis Index is included in the WHO basic oral health survey methods.[15] Dental fluorosis has been classified in a number of other ways, including the Tooth Surface Index of Fluorosis, the Thylstrup-Fejerskov Index, and the Fluorosis Risk Index.[16, 17]

Access to Oral Health Services

Access to Community Prevention: Water Fluoridation

Community water fluoridation, a community preventive service, is measured by the percentage of persons served by public water systems containing optimally fluoridated water.[31] Optimal levels of fluoridation are achieved by adjusting fluoride to obtain a concentration between 0.7 and 1.2 parts per million (ppm). The optimal fluoride concentration is determined by geographical areas based on mean daily temperature; thus, states have different levels of optimal concentration of fluoride in water.

To characterize a community as optimally fluoridated, it is necessary to compare tap water or water samples from water treatment plants with the level determined by the state to be optimal for that community. The Water Fluoridation Reporting System (WFRS) by the Division of Oral Health, CDC, monitors what the state health agencies have reported as the optimal level for each public water system within the state.[4] These reports are compiled for a census.

See Table 4–1 for a summary of the ways in which community water fluoridation will be monitored for *Healthy People 2010*.

Access to the Oral Health Care System

Access to the oral health system consists of many facets, including availability, accessibility, accommodation, affordability, and acceptability.[32] Multiple factors have been assessed to explain the use of clinical oral health services. These factors have been summarized as epidemiologic, social, demographic, personal, and psychological, as well as characteristic of the oral health care system.[3]

A common measure of access to and utilization of the oral health care system is having an annual dental visit. This measure is assessed by determining the length of time since the last visit to a dentist or dental clinic. See Table 4–1 for a summary of the ways in which use of the oral health care system will be monitored for *Healthy People 2010*.

Responses to interview questions have been used to measure the percentage of persons who have had a dental visit in the past year. The National Health Interview Survey, which uses a face-to-face interview to measure dental visits, is used to measure progress of the *Healthy People 2010* objectives regarding dental attendance. Other national surveys, such as the NHANES and Medical Expenditure Panel Survey (MEPS), use face-to-face interviews with structured questionnaires to evaluate dental visits. Specific questions about dental visits are included in these questionnaires.

The CDC, through its state-specific **Behavioral Risk Factor Surveillance Survey (BRFSS)**, conducts telephone interviews to assess dental attendance. In addition, self-administered questionnaires have been used by states and localities to determine access to dental care. The questionnaire may be completed by adult participants in surveys or by parents of children participating in school-based oral health surveys. The National Nursing Home Survey, conducted by the CDC in 1997, measured the receipt of dental services by nursing home residents.

Other important measures associated with access to oral care include the following:

- Dental attendance for routine check-ups or cleanings
- Assessment of dental insurance coverage
- Usual source of dental care
- Reason for not having a dental visit in the past year
- Difficulty in obtaining needed dental care
- Purpose of last dental visit

Figure 4–2 outlines examples of questions about access to care that are included with the Basic Screening Survey methods in the Screening

1. During the past 6 months, did {you/your child} have a toothache more than once, when biting or chewing? [Source: National Health Interview Survey, 1989]

1. Yes
2. No
3. Don't know/don't remember

2. About how long has it been since {you/your child} last visited a dentist? Include all types of dentists, such as orthodontists, oral surgeons, and all other dental specialists, as well as dental hygienists. [Source: National Health Interview Survey, 1997]

1. 6 months or less
2. More than 6 months, but not more than 1 year ago
3. More than 1 year ago, but not more than 3 years ago
4. More than 3 years ago
5. Never have been
6. Don't know/don't remember

3. What was the main reason that {you/your child} last visited a dentist? (Please check one.) [Source: National Health Interview Survey,1986]

1. Went in on own for check-up, examination, or cleaning
2. Was called in by the dentist for check-up, examination, or cleaning
3. Something was wrong, bothering, or hurting
4. Went for treatment of a condition that dentist discovered at earlier check-up or examination
5. Other
6. Don't know/don't remember

4. During the past 12 months, was there a time when {you/your child} needed dental care but could not get it at that time? [Source: National Health Interview Survey, 1994]

1. Yes
2. No
3. Don't know/don't remember

5. The last time {you/your child} could not get the dental care (you/he/she) needed, what was the main reason (you/he/she) couldn't get care? (Please check one.) [Source: National Health Interview Survey, 1994]

1. Could not afford it
2. No insurance
3. Dentist did not accept Medicaid/insurance
4. Not serious enough
5. Wait too long in clinic/office
6. Difficulty in getting appointment
7. Don't like/trust/believe in dentists
8. No dentist available
9. Didn't know where to go
10. No way to get there
11. Hours not convenient
12. Speak a different language
13. Health of another family member
14. Other reason
15. Don't know/don't remember

6. Do you have any kind of insurance that pays for some or all of {you/your child's} MEDICAL OR SURGICAL CARE? Include health insurance obtained through employment or purchased directly as well as government program like Medicaid.

1. Yes
2. No
3. Don't know/don't remember

Figure 4-2. Questions to evaluate the use of the oral health care system. (Adapted from Association of State and Territorial Dental Directors: Basic Screening Surveys: An Approach to Monitoring Community Oral Health. Screening Training Project, 1999.[9])

Illustration continued on following page

7. Do you have any kind of insurance that pays for some or all of {your/ your child's} DENTAL CARE? Include health insurance obtained through employment or purchased directly as well as government programs like Medicaid.

1. Yes
2. No
3. Don't know/don't remember

Additional questions for survey planners to consider:

8. During the past 12 months, was there a time when you felt that {you/your child} needed MEDICAL CARE OR SURGERY but could not get it at that time? [Source: Modified from National Health Interview Survey, 1994]

1. Yes
2. No
3. Don't know/don't remember

9. The last time {you/your child} could not get the MEDICAL CARE OR SURGERY {you/he/she} needed, what was the main reason (you/he/she) couldn't get care? [Source: National Health Interview Survey, 1994]

1. Could not afford it
2. No insurance
3. Doctor did not accept Medicaid/insurance
4. Not serious enough
5. Wait too long in clinic/office
6. Difficulty in getting appointment
7. Don't like/trust/believe in doctors
8. No doctor available
9. Didn't know where to go
10. No way to get there
11. Hours not convenient
12. Speak a different language
13. Health of another family member
14. Other reason
15. Don't know/don't remember

For all questions, refused/no response is a coding option but is not listed as a choice on the questionnaire. For one-digit variables, 9 is coded. For two-digit variables, the refused/no response code is 99.

Figure 4–2. *Continued*

Training Project, developed by the ASTTD.[9] These questions can be included in a self-administered questionnaire or can be asked during a telephone or face-to-face interview.

Measurement of Oral Health, Well-being, and Quality of Life

A better understanding of cultural, social, behavioral, psychological, and economic factors related to oral conditions and treatments can contribute to oral health efforts at the community level.[33, 34] During an assessment, it is also important to consider the belief systems as well as cultural values, customs, traditions, and institutions related to oral health of individuals and groups.[3] Measurements of knowledge, attitudes, beliefs, and behaviors have traditionally been used to evaluate personal oral health practices and use of the oral health care system.[1, 3]

Data collection methods have been developed to assess oral health knowledge, attitudes, beliefs, and behaviors. Multiple measurements have been designed to evaluate diverse factors as they relate to oral health care–seeking behaviors, oral hygiene and home care practices, dietary practices, use of tobacco and alcohol, age-appropriate safety measures, and use of protective gear.[1]

The development of sociodental indicators has been advocated to assess the nonclinical aspects of oral diseases.[3] Measures have been recommended to document the full impact of oral disorders and treatment within populations. Different measures have been used to evaluate economic impact as well as social and psychological consequences of oral diseases, conditions, and injuries. These measures have been developed to assess outcomes at the individual and societal levels. The term *oral health–related quality of life* has been adopted as a construct that considers multiple dimensions of oral health.[35]

Perceived health status and general assessment of oral health are common measurements used in population-based oral health surveys. These questions were included in the International Collaborative Study of Oral Health Outcomes, sponsored by WHO.[36] The questions use a basic Likert measurement scale to assess self-perceived health status:

- Would you describe your general health as excellent, very good, good, fair, poor, or very poor?
- How would you describe the health of your teeth and gums? Is it excellent, very good, good, fair, poor, or very poor?

Satisfaction with oral health status is another measurement used in surveys. Assessment instruments such the Geriatric Oral Health Assessment Instrument (GOHAI) and the Oral Health Impact Profile (OHIP) have been developed to evaluate oral health–related quality of life.[1, 35]

The psychosocial and functional dimensions of oral health have been used in studies of population groups.[1, 34] These dimensions consider the crucial sensory, communicative, gustatory, and psychosocial functions of the structures related to the teeth, mouth, and face, such as social function, and the impact of oral disorders on intimacy, personal contact, social integration, and social roles.[1]

The functional dimensions of oral health have been assessed and include measurements of self-perceived oral functional status and well-being, including self-reported evaluations of tooth loss, oral pain, eating ability, and ability to sleep. The impact of oral symptoms and pain can also be included in assessments.

Self-reported evaluations can assess presence or absence of pain in the teeth or soft tissues of the mouth from acute or chronic oral pain, dental pain, and facial pain. In addition, studies have considered social response to facial appearance by assessing social and psychological outcomes of malocclusion, craniofacial anomalies, and oral cancer. Such assessments can include measurements of self-concept, psychosocial development, and social perceptions.

Economic dimensions include indirect and direct economic impacts of oral health problems and their treatments.[1] A measurement of indirect economic impacts is self-reported reductions in normal activities related to dental conditions and dental attendance.[1] Answers to questions in a structured questionnaire can evaluate work-loss days, school-loss days, re-duced activity days, and bed days due to acute dental conditions and dental visit. This measure is included in the National Health Interview Survey. Years of life lost can be calculated on the basis of premature deaths from oral and pharyngeal cancer.[1]

Direct economic impacts include direct costs related to dental and oral problems for society and individuals. In addition, analyses of cost benefit and cost effectiveness can be made for preventive and therapeutic treat-ments to evaluate direct economic impacts of oral health problems and their treatments.

Measures of oral health, well-being, and quality of life can be used to demonstrate the significance of oral health conditions for individuals as well as society as a whole. It helps to ensure that treatments provided re-sult in health gains that enhance not only the individual's clinical status but also his or her psychological well-being. Assessing social, psychologi-cal, and economic impacts can be used to identify population subgroups and oral diseases that need to be targeted for health promotion and dis-ease prevention efforts.[1]

Measurement of Infrastructure, Capacity, and Resources

Infrastructure, capacity, and resources are key elements by which states and localities can effectively address oral health problems.[7]

Infrastructure consists of systems, people, relationships, and resources that enable states and localities to perform public health functions and address oral health problems. Within a public health agency, infrastruc-ture includes assessment, surveillance, information systems, planning, policy development, applied research, training, standards development, quality management, coordination, and systems of care.

Capacity enables the development of expertise and competence and the implementation of strategies.

Resources include personnel and financial capital as well as available time. The public health and personal health work force must have the necessary capacity and expertise to effectively address oral health prob-lems and issues in jurisdictions and states.[10]

See Table 4–1 for a summary of the ways in which infrastructure and ca-pacity of the oral health system will be monitored for *Healthy People 2010.*

To ensure achievement of the *Healthy People 2010* oral health objectives, it is necessary that instruments and methods be developed to assess the current status, best practices, and future development of infrastructure, capacity, and resources necessary to improve oral health at state and local levels. States and localities that can evaluate and develop these key elements will be better prepared to maintain fully effective essential public health services for oral health and to achieve the oral health objectives.

STATUS OF ORAL HEALTH IN THE UNITED STATES

In the United States, progress has been made in reducing the extent and severity of common oral diseases.[1] Over the past 50 years, major improvements in oral health have been seen nationally for many Americans, yet oral diseases remain common and widespread in the United States. Oral diseases and conditions still afflict most people at some time throughout their life span. Safe and effective measures of preventing oral diseases exist but are underused. Effective preventive measures include (1) community water fluoridation, (2) application of dental sealants, (3) regular dental care, and (4) tobacco cessation. Preventive measures need to be adopted and applied by communities, individuals, and professionals to ensure marked improvements of the nation's oral health in the future.[1]

SOCIAL IMPACT OF ORAL DISEASES

Oral diseases are progressive and cumulative and become more complex over time. They can jeopardize physical growth, development, self-concept, and the capacity to learn. They influence eating and communicating. Oral diseases affect economic productivity and compromise a person's ability to work at home or on the job or to concentrate in school.

The social impact of oral disease in children is substantial. More than 51 million school hours are lost each year as a result of dental problems.[1] Poor children experience nearly 12 times more restricted activity days than do their counterparts from higher-income families. Among those who lost school time, youngsters from low-income families, members of minority communities, and families without insurance missed more hours.[37] Children with early childhood caries—oftentimes a severe and painful form of dental caries—can demonstrate failure to thrive and be underweight.[38] Serious lifetime functional, aesthetic, and social consequences can be outcomes for children and adults with severe developmental and acquired oral and facial conditions.[1] The CDC estimated that 16.2 years of life were lost per person who died prematurely from oral and pharyngeal cancer.[1] This figure exceeds the average 15.4 years lost for all cancer sites.

Dental diseases in adults affect their economic productivity and compromise their ability to get jobs. Employed American adults lose more than 164 million hours of work each year because of dental disease or dental visits.[1] Among those who missed work, women, African Americans, low wage earners, employees with less education, and the uninsured miss the greatest number of hours. Employees of service industries loose from 2 to 3.5 times more hours of work than hours lost by executives or professional workers.[37]

Oral and dental diseases influence an individual's ability to eat, communicate, and interact in society. For example, a WHO-supported study found that among Navajo schoolchildren living in parts of the Navajo reservation in Arizona and New Mexico, 25% avoided laughing or smiling and 20% avoided meeting other people because of the way their teeth looked.[36] As a consequence of dental pain, almost 25% of Navajo adults were unable to chew hard foods and nearly 20% reported difficulty sleeping.[36]

BURDEN OF ORAL DISEASES AND DISORDERS

Despite improvements in oral health status, profound disparities remain in specific population groups. For some oral diseases and conditions, the magnitude of the differences in oral health status among population groups is striking.[1] The burden of oral diseases is spread unevenly throughout the population. People who experience the worst oral health are found among the poor of all ages, with poor children and poor older Americans particularly vulnerable.[1] Members of racial and ethnic minorities experience a disproportionate level of oral health problems. People who are medically compromised or who have disabilities are at greater risk for oral disease; in turn, oral diseases further jeopardize their overall health and well-being. This burden of oral disease restricts activities in school, work, and home and often significantly diminishes quality of life.

The following text provides a broad overview of the current **status** and **trends** associated with oral health in the United States. It concentrates on the oral health indicators included in *Healthy People 2010*. These indicators can provide a framework for oral health assessments at the state and local levels. Table 4–2 reviews the national trends and targets of key oral health indicators in the United States.

CURRENT STATUS AND TRENDS

Dental Caries

Children and Adolescents

Despite a tremendous decline in dental caries in children in the United States since the 1950s, tooth decay remains the single most common chronic disease of childhood.[1] It is five times more common than asthma and seven times more common than hay fever.[1]

Text continued on page 110

Table 4–2						
Oral Health in the United States:						
National Trends and Targets*						
Oral Health Indicator	**Age (yr)/ Location**	**Baseline Data (for HP 2000 Target)**	**HP 2000 Target**	**Final Data for HP 2000 Target (Baseline for HP 2010 Target)**	**Summary (Attainment of HP 2000 Target)**	**HP 2010 Target**
Dental Caries Experience						
Reduce dental caries in young children (primary teeth)	2–4	—	—	18%	—	11%
Reduce dental caries in children (primary or permanent teeth)	6–8	54%	35%	52%	Progress	42%
Reduce dental caries in adolescents (permanent teeth)	15	78%	60%	61%	Progress	51%
Untreated Dental Decay						
Reduce untreated dental decay in young children (primary teeth)	2–4	—	—	16%	—	9%
Reduce untreated dental decay in children (primary or permanent teeth)	6–8	28%	20%	29%	Reversed	21%
Reduce untreated dental decay in adolescents (permanent teeth)	15	24%	15%	20%	Progress	15%
Reduce untreated dental decay in adults	35–44	—	—	27%	—	15%

Table continued on following page

				Final Data for HP 2000 Target		
Oral Health Indicator	**Age (yr)/ Location**	**Baseline Data (for HP 2000 Target)**	**HP 2000 Target**	**(Baseline for HP 2010 Target)**	**Summary (Attainment of HP 2000 Target)**	**HP 2010 Target**
No Permanent Tooth Loss						
Increase adults who have never lost a permanent tooth	35–44	31%	45%	31%	No change	42%
Complete Tooth Loss						
Reduce adults who have lost all their teeth	65+	36%	20%	30%	Progress	
Reduce adults who have lost all their teeth	65–74	—	—	26%	—	20%
Reduce Periodontal Disease						
Reduce gingivitis among adults	35–44	41%	30%	48%	Reversed	41%
Reduce destructive periodontal disease	35–44	25%	15%	22%	Progress	14%
Reduce Oral and Pharyngeal Cancer Deaths (Age-adjusted rate per 100,000)						
Reduce oral and pharyngeal cancer deaths in males	45–74	13.6	10.5	10.3	Met	—
Reduce oral and pharyngeal cancer deaths in females	45–74	4.8	4.1	3.5	Met	—
Reduce oral and pharyngeal cancer deaths	All ages	—	—	2.9	—	2.6

Table 4–2
**Oral Health in the United States:
National Trends and Targets*** (Continued)

				Table 4–2		
			Oral Health in the United States:			
			National Trends and Targets* (*Continued*)			

Oral Health Indicator	Age (yr)/ Location	Baseline Data (for HP 2000 Target)	HP 2000 Target	Final Data for HP 2000 Target (Baseline for HP 2010 Target)	Summary (Attainment of HP 2000 Target)	HP 2010 Target
Early Detection of Oral and Pharyngeal Cancer						
Increase early detection of oral and pharyngeal cancer	All ages	—	—	35%	—	50%
Annual Examinations for Oral and Pharyngeal Cancer						
Increase annual examinations for oral and pharyngeal cancer (age-adjusted)	40+	—	—	14%	—	35%
Dental Sealants						
Increase dental sealants in children	8	11%	50%	23%	Progress	50%
Increase dental sealants in adolescents	14	8%	50%	24%	Progress	50%
Community Water Fluoridation						
Increase no. of persons on public water system receiving fluoridated water	All ages	61%	75%	62%	Progress	75%

Table continued on following page

				Table 4–2		
			Oral Health in the United States:			
			National Trends and Targets* (Continued)			

Oral Health Indicator	Age (yr)/ Location	Baseline Data (for HP 2000 Target)	HP 2000 Target	Final Data for HP 2000 Target (Baseline for HP 2010 Target)	Summary (Attainment of HP 2000 Target)	HP 2010 Target
Use of Oral Health Care System (Annual dental visit age-adjusted)						
Increase oral health screening, referral, follow-up first-time school attendees, at first school experience	5	66%	90%	75%	Progress	83%
Increase use of oral health care system by adults	35+	54%	70%	63%	Progress	—
Increase use of oral health care system by children and adults	>2	—	—	65%	—	83%
Increase use of dental services by low-income children	<19	—	—	20%	—	57%
Use of Oral Health Care System by Residents in Long-Term Care Facilities						
For long-term care, oral examination and services provided within 90 days	No data	100%	No data	—	—	
Increase use of oral health care system by residents in long-term care facilities	—	—	19%	—	25%	

Oral Health Indicator	Age (yr)/ Location	Baseline Data (for HP 2000 Target)	HP 2000 Target	Final Data for HP 2000 Target (Baseline for HP 2010 Target)	Summary (Attainment of HP 2000 Target)	HP 2010 Target
Preventive Strategies						
Increase topical/ systemic fluorides among nonfluoridated areas	All ages	50%	85%	No data	No data	—
Increase caregivers using feeding practices that prevent early childhood caries	All ages	55%	75%	No data	No data	—
Extend use of protective head, face, eye, and mouth equipment	All ages	No data	No data	No data	No data	—
Smokeless Tobacco Use						
Reduce smokeless tobacco use among males	12–17	6.6%	4%	3.7%	Met	1% (Grades 9–12)†
Reduce smokeless tobacco use among males	18–24	8.9%	4%	6.9%	Progress	0.4% (>18 yr)†
School-Based Health Centers with Oral Health Component (Developmental Objective)	All centers	—	—	Data not collected	—	Data not collected
Health Centers with Oral Health Components (Developmental Objective)	All centers	—	—	34%	—	75%

Table continued on following page

				Final Data for HP 2000 Target		
		Baseline Data		(Baseline	Summary	
	Age	(for HP	HP	for HP	(Attainment	HP
Oral Health	(yr)/	2000	2000	2010	of HP 2000	2010
Indicator	Location	Target)	Target	Target)	Target)	Target
(Referral for Cleft Lip or Palate) Increase states with system for recording and referring orofacial clefts	All states and D.C.	11 states	40 states	23 states and D.C.	Progress	50 states and D.C.
State-Based Surveillance System	All states and D.C.	—	—	0	—	50 states and D.C.
Tribal, State, and Local Agencies	Specific jurisdictions	—	—	Data not collected	—	Data not collected

Table 4–2

Oral Health in the United States: National Trends and Targets* (Continued)

* Table includes oral health measures from *Healthy People 2000* (*HP 2000*) and *Healthy People 2010* (*HP 2010*).
† See Reference 4, tobacco use chapter, for specific *HP 2010* targets.
Data from Centers for Disease Control and Prevention: Healthy People 2000 Review, 1999–2000. Hyattsville, Md, Public Health Service, 1999[31]; and Healthy People 2010: Understanding and Improving Health (Conference ed, 2 vols). Washington, DC, U.S. Department of Health and Human Services, 2000.[4]

The average number of decayed and filled teeth (dft) among 2- to 4-year-olds has remained unchanged over the past 25 years.[4] According to NHANES III, 18% of young children 2 to 4 years of age experienced dental caries in their primary dentition during the years 1988 to 1994.[4] Of these children, 16% had untreated caries in their primary teeth. Eighty-two percent of these children in 1988 to 1994 were free of caries.

Early childhood caries affects the primary teeth of infants and young children 1 to 5 years of age.[4] Sometimes referred to as baby bottle tooth decay or nursing caries, it can be a devastating condition, often requiring thousands of dollars and a hospital visit with general anesthesia during treatment.[39] Substantial pain, psychological stress, health risks, and expense are associated with restorative care for children affected by early childhood caries.[40] Infant feeding practices, in which children are put to bed with formula or other sweetened drinks and fall asleep while feeding, have been associated with this condition.[40]

Minority children aged 2 to 4 years in the United States have more dental caries than white children[4]:

- ◆ Young African American children, 1.6 times more
- ◆ Young Mexican American children, 2.1 times more
- ◆ Young Asian children, 2.3 times more
- ◆ Young Native American children, 5 times more

America's youngest and poorest young children, aged 2 to 4 years and living below the poverty level, have almost three times as much dental caries as in children of higher-income families (>200% poverty).[31] Almost 80% of cases of dental caries remain untreated in young poor children.[41]

The prevalence of dental caries in the permanent dentition of school-aged children has been declining in the United States over the past two decades. This decline is the result of various preventive measures, such as community water fluoridation and increased use of fluoride toothpastes and mouth rinses.[1] Despite this reduction, more than one half (52%) of children aged 6 to 8 years experienced dental caries in their primary or permanent teeth in the years 1988 to 1994.[4] This proportion had decreased only slightly from 54% in the years 1986 to 1987.[32]

The proportion of untreated dental caries in school-aged children also has been declining overall but has increased among children aged 6 to 8 years. Nearly one third (29%) of 6- to 8-year-olds had untreated dental caries in 1988 to 1994, up in 28% in 1986 to 1987.[31] In the years 1988 to 1994, by the third grade 60% of students had experienced tooth decay and 30% of these third-graders had untreated dental caries.[4]

Caries experience is cumulative, thus higher among adolescents than among young children.[4] By age 15 years, two thirds (61%) of teenagers had experienced dental caries in their permanent dentition, according to a national survey in 1988 to 1994.[4] Thirty-nine percent of these teens were caries-free. In comparison, 78% of adolescents during the period 1986 to 1987 had experienced dental caries.[31] In the years 1988 to 1994, 20% of teens 15 years of age had untreated tooth decay and were in need of treatment.[4] This proportion has decreased slightly from 24% of teens with untreated dental caries in the period 1986 to 1987.[31] By the time students finish high school, about 80% have experienced dental caries.[4]

As with general health, oral health status in the United States tends to vary on the basis of social and demographic factors. Dental caries, however, remains a significant problem in specific populations, particularly poor children and adults from certain racial and ethnic groups.[1, 4] Most tooth decay is experienced by only a few children. National data indicate that 80% of cases of dental caries in permanent teeth are now concentrated in only 25% of school-aged children (5 to 17 years old).[18]

Children from minority racial and ethnic groups (e.g., American Indian, Alaska Native, Asian or Pacific Islander, Mexican American, and black or African American), whose parents have less than a high school education or who have a low income are often markedly at increased risk for dental caries.[4, 31] For example, the level of untreated dental caries among African American children aged 6 to 8 years (36%) and Mexican American children (43%) is greater than for white children (26%).[4] A statewide oral health survey in California found 69% of Asian or Pacific Islander children 6 to 8 years of age had dental caries in the years 1993 to 1994.[4] In 1999, the oral health survey of Native Americans reported that 71% American Indian or Alaska Native children 6 to 8 years of age had untreated dental caries.[4] Disparities in the frequency of dental caries among children are shown in Table 4–3.

Young and Older Adults

Of all adults 18 years of age and older, 85% have experienced dental caries.[1] More than 37% of persons aged 65 years or older in the United States with teeth had at least one decayed or filled root surface.[2] Also, 50% of people 75 years and older had root caries affecting at least one tooth.[1] Approximately 27% of adults 35 to 44 years of age had untreated dental caries in 1988 to

Table 4–3

Disparities in Dental Caries and Dental Sealants

Disparity	Age (yr)	All	Race/Ethnicity			Family Income*			Level of Education†		
			White	Black	Hispanic/ Mexican American	Poor	Near- Poor	Mid- High	<HS	HS	>HS
Dental caries	2–4	18%	15%	24%	27%	29%	21%	10%	29%	18%	12%
(*ever* had	6–8	52%	51%	50%	68%	62%	60%	42%	65%	52%	43%
tooth	15	61%	60%	70%	57%	77%	69%	51%	59%	63%	61%
decay											
experience)											
Dental caries	2–4	16%	11%	22%	24%	26%	20%	7%	26%	16%	9%
(has	6–8	29%	26%	36%	43%	47%	32%	16%	44%	30%	25%
untreated	15	20%	19%	29%	27%	20%	28%	16%	29%	18%	15%
tooth decay	35–44	27%	24%	47%	34%	NA	NA	NA	51%	34%	16%
now)	15	20%	19%	29%	27%	20%	28%	16%	29%	18%	15%
Dental	8	23%	26%	11%	7%	3%	18%	35%	17%	12%	35%
sealants											
(1st molar	14	24%	28%	5%	7%	12%	11%	39%	4%	17%	42%
only)											
(1st and	14	15%	19%	5%	7%	NA	NA	NA	NA	NA	NA
2nd											
molar)											

* Family income is defined as poor, <100% FPL (Federal Poverty Level); near-poor, 100% to 199% FPL; mid-high income, >200% FPL.
† Level of education (high school [HS]) is defined as that of head of household.
Data from National Health and Nutrition Examination Survey (NHANES), 1988–1994.
Adapted from Centers for Disease Control and Prevention, Healthy People 2000 Review, 1999–2000. Hyattsville, Md, Public Health Service, 1999.[31]

1994.[4] Untreated dental caries can lead to pain, abscess, extensive dental treatment, and extraction of the tooth, and dental care can be quite costly. As the trends in aging continue, adults will lose fewer teeth as they age but will have more teeth that are at risk for dental caries throughout life.[4]

Findings from the NHANES III survey showed disparities in dental caries among adults, with twice as many young African American adults (47%) as white adults (24%) affected by dental caries.[4] More than three times as many of these young adults (35 to 44 years of age) with less than a high school education (51%) had untreated dental caries than did adults with some college education (16%).[4] Disparities in the frequency of dental caries among adults are shown in Table 4–3.

Dental Sealants

Dental sealants can be very effective in preventing dental caries on the pit and fissure surfaces of teeth, but few children receive them. The percentage of school-aged children with dental sealants has risen among specific groups in recent years as the public and private sectors increasingly use the procedure, dental insurance pays for dental sealants, and parents request sealants for their children.[42] Despite the effectiveness of dental sealants, fewer than 25% of children in the United States have received them.[4] Great disparities in the use of dental sealants are found among children based on race and ethnicity, family income, and parental education.[4] These striking disparities are shown in Table 4–3.

As few as 3% of poor 8-year old children have had dental sealants, in contrast to 35% of children from families with higher income levels. Only 7% of Hispanic children aged 8 years and 11% of their African American peers have had dental sealants. In 1990, the National Health Interview Survey found that 23% of adults in the United States reported that dental sealants prevented dental caries.[43] Hispanic adults (12%), African American (12%) adults, and adults with less than a high school education were less likely to know the purpose of dental sealants than non-Hispanic (26%) and white (25%) adults.[43]

Community Water Fluoridation

Community water fluoridation, a cornerstone community preventive service in the United States, has been a major factor in the decline of dental caries. Fluoridation of water supplies grew rapidly from its inception in 1945 until about 1980. Since then, the increase has been lower in recent years.[44] The proportion of the population living in communities with fluoridated water supplies has reached 62%.[44] About 100 million persons still lack access to the benefits of community water fluoridation.

According to a national survey of adults in 1998, 70% of respondents indicated that water supplies should be fluoridated in communities.[45] In 1990, only 62% of adults had recognized that the primary purpose of water fluoridation is to prevent dental caries. Persons with lower levels of education, Hispanic adults, and African American adults were less likely to know the purpose of water fluoridation.[46] When asked to identify the best method of preventing dental caries, only 7% of adults considered fluoride the correct answer and 70% indicated tooth brushing and flossing to be the most effective.[43]

Periodontal Disease

During the period 1988 to 1994, nearly half (48%) of adults aged 35 to 44 years had gingivitis (inflammation of the gums).[4] This figure represents an increase from the 41% of young adults with gingivitis in 1985 to 1986.[31] Gingivitis will probably remain a substantial problem and may increase as tooth loss from dental caries declines or may result from the use of some systemic medications.[4]

Destructive periodontal disease (defined as loss of attachment of 4 mm or greater) affected 22% of dentate adults 35 to 44 years of age in 1988 to 1994.[4] The incidence of this problem declined among young adults from 25% in 1985 to 1986.[31] Severe periodontal disease (defined as 6 mm of loss of attachment) affects 14% of adults aged 45 to 54 years and 23% of adults aged 65 to 74 years. Destructive periodontal disease seems to increase with age.[1]

Gingivitis occurs frequently among American Indians or Alaska Natives, Mexican Americans, adults with low incomes, and adults with less than a high school education.[1] Among certain population groups, the prevalence of destructive periodontal disease is higher, for example, among 35- to 44-year-old men, American Indians or Alaska Natives, African American adults, adults with low family incomes, and adults with less than a high school education.[4] At all ages, more severe periodontal disease is seen among males and adults at the lowest income levels.[1] Disparities in adult periodontal health related to income, education, race, and ethnicity are summarized in Table 4–4.

Tooth Loss

Fewer adults are undergoing tooth extraction because of dental caries or periodontal disease. The percentage of people who have lost all of their natural teeth has been declining over the past 50 years.[1] Of adults 35 to 44 years of age, 31% had never lost a permanent tooth during the period 1988 to 1994, although this oral health indicator has not changed since the mid-1980s.[31]

Approximately 26% of the American population aged 65 to 74 years are edentulous (i.e., have lost all of their natural teeth). Among persons aged 65 to 74 years in 1997, 39% of persons with less than a high school education were edentulous, compared with 13% of persons with at least some college.[4] In this same age group, edentulousness is also higher among older African American (30%) than among Hispanic (24%) and white (25%) older adults.[4] Disparities related to tooth loss are shown in Table 4–5.

Table 4–4
Adults: Disparities in Periodontal Disease

Disparity	Age (yr)	All	Race/Ethnicity			Family Income*			Level of Education†		
			White	Black	Hispanic/ Mexican American	Poor	Near-Poor	Mid-High	<HS	HS	>HS
Gingivitis	35–44	48%	47%	51%	64%	66%	45%	23%	60%	52%	42%
Destructive periodontal disease	35–44	22%	20%	33%	24%	42%	31%	17%	35%	28%	15%

* Family income is defined as poor, <100% FPL (Federal Poverty Level); near-poor, 100% to 199% FPL; mid-high income, >200% FPL.
  † Level of education (high school [HS]) is defined as that of head of household.
  Data from National Health and Nutrition Examination Survey (NHANES), 1988–1994.
  Adapted from Centers for Disease Control and Prevention, Healthy People 2000 Review, 1999–2000. Hyattsville, Md, Public Health Service, 1999.[31]

Oral and Pharyngeal Cancer

Oral and pharyngeal cancers include different malignant tumors that affect the oral cavity and pharynx. Most of these tumors are squamous cell carcinomas.[47] These may include cancers of the lip, tongue, floor of the mouth, palate, gingival and alveolar mucosa, buccal mucosa, and oropharynx.

The American Cancer Society has reported that in the United States, 30,200 people are found to have oral and pharyngeal cancers and 7800 persons die of these cancers each year.[48] These cancers occurs more frequently than leukemia, Hodgkin's disease, and cancers of the brain, cervix, ovary, liver, pancreas, bone, thyroid gland, testes, and stomach.

Table 4–5
Adults: Disparities in Loss of Teeth

Disparity	Age (yr)	All	Race/Ethnicity			Family Income*			Level of Education†		
			White	Black	Hispanic/ Mexican American	Poor	Near-Poor	Mid-High	<HS	HS	>HS
No tooth loss‡	35–44	31%	34%	12%	23%	17%	18%	36%	18%	28%	58%
Complete	65–74	26%	25%	30%	24%	NA	NA	NA	39%	26%	13%
tooth loss§	75+	30%	NA	NA	NA	46%	44%	NA	NA	NA	NA

* Family income is defined as poor, <100% FPL (Federal Poverty Level); near-poor, 100% to 199% FPL; mid-high income, >200% FPL.
  † Level of education (high school [HS]) is defined as that of head of household.
  ‡ Data from National Health and Nutrition Examination Survey (NHANES), 1988–1994.
  § Data from National Health Interview Survey, 1997.
  Adapted from Centers for Disease Control and Prevention, Healthy People 2000 Review, 1999–2000. Hyattsville, Md, Public Health Service, 1999.[31]

The occurrence of oral and pharyngeal cancers varies by race and ethnicity. African Americans and whites have 12.5 and 10.0 new cases per 100,000 per year, respectively, whereas Asians and Pacific Islanders, Hispanics, and American Indian and Alaska Natives have 7.9, 6.4, and 5.8 new cases per year, respectively.[49] For adult men 45 to 74 years of age, the mortality rate increases to 20.6 for African Americans and 10.3 for white males.[31] Table 4–6 compares the disparities related to oral and pharyngeal cancers.

In the United States, oral and pharyngeal cancers constitute the fourth most common cancer among African American men, the seventh most common cancer among white men, and the 14th most common among women.[49] The median age at diagnosis of oral and pharyngeal cancer is 64 years, and the rate of occurrence increases with age.

The 5-year survival rates for oral and pharyngeal cancers have remained unchanged since the early 1960s.[50] The rate is only 52%, and most of these cancers are diagnosed at late stages.[50] In only 35% of all individuals with oral and pharyngeal cancers is the diagnosis made at an early stage (21% for African American men, 36% for Hispanic men, and 38% for white men).[36]

African American men have experienced increases in both death rates and new case rates, and their 5-year survival rate is much poorer than that for whites (31% versus 55%).[48, 50] African American men suffer the highest incidence of and the lowest survival rates from oral and pharyngeal cancers. At every stage of diagnosis, the survival rate for African Americans is lower than that for whites.[50]

Tobacco use is the major risk factor for oral and pharyngeal cancers, accounting for more than 90% of cases in the United States.[51] In 1998, 24% of adults smoked cigarettes, 2.5% smoked cigars, and nearly 3% used smokeless ("spit") tobacco. Forty percent of students (grades 9–12) reported using tobacco; of these students, 35% smoked cigarettes, 18% smoked cigars, and 8% used spit tobacco.[52]

Overall levels of knowledge about risk factors for oral cancer are low. There is extensive misinformation and a general lack of knowledge among American adults about the signs, symptoms, and risk factors for oral and pharyngeal cancers. According to the National Health Interview Survey in 1990, this gap in knowledge was present across race, ethnic groups, and frequency of recent visits for dental and medical care. In 1990, only 25% of adults in the United States could identify one sign of oral cancer.[53] Tobacco use was the only risk factor most adults identified correctly. There was a lower level of knowledge of other risk factors across all racial and ethnic groups of American adults. Only 36% of adults knew that excessive exposure to sunlight definitely increased the risk of lip cancer.

Only 15% of adults in the United States reported ever having an oral cancer examination; of these, 48% of adults aged 40 years and older indicated having had an oral cancer examination in the past year, according to the National Health Interview Survey in 1992.[54] Respondents most likely to have had an oral cancer examination included those above the poverty level, those who were white, those who were non-Hispanic, those who were 40 to 65 years of age, those who had more than a high school

Table 4–6
Adults: Disparities in Oral Cancer

Disparity		Age (yr)	All	Race/Ethnicity		
				White	Black	Hispanic/ Mexican American
Oral cancer	Males	45–74		10.3	20.6	NA
mortality rate*	Females	45–74		3.5	5.1	NA
Percentage diagnosed at earliest stage of oral cancer†			35%	38%	21%	36%
Receipt of oral cancer examination‡		>40	7%	8%	3%	8%

* Data from National Medical Expediture Panel Survey, 1996, Agency for Health Care Policy and Research. Oral cancer rate per 100,000.
† Data from Surveillance, Epidemiology, and End Results (SEER) Program, 1996.
‡ Data from National Health Interview Survey, 1992, Centers for Disease Control and Prevention, National Center for Health Statistics.
Adapted from Centers for Disease Control and Prevention, Healthy People 2000 Review, 1999–2000. Hyattsville, Md, Public Health Service, 1999.[31]

education, and those who had a higher level of knowledge about risk factors for oral cancer. See Table 4–6 for a comparison of the disparities related to oral and pharyngeal cancers based on race and ethnicity.

Other Oral Conditions

Cleft Lip and/or Palate

Cleft lip with or without cleft palate is one of the more common birth defects in the United States. This congenital defect occurs in about 1 per 1000 live births and affects approximately 1 of 600 live births in whites and 1 of 1850 live births in African Americans.[29] States should have an efficient mechanism in place for identifying, recording, and referring infants with oral clefts for treatment. Of 50 states plus the District of Columbia, 23 reported referral and reporting systems for persons with a cleft lip and/or palate.[4] Care by a multidisciplinary team has been shown to be an effective approach in providing services for people with craniofacial anomalies.

Malocclusion

In a national survey, it was found that 9% of persons 8 to 50 years of age had severe crowding of the anterior incisors and 25% had no crowding.[27] Approximately 9% of persons had a posterior crossbite; this condition was most common in non-Hispanic whites. Severe overbite was found in 8%, and a similar percentage had a severe overjet. Fewer than 5% of non-Hispanic whites had an open bite.

Orofacial Injuries

Injuries to the head, face, and teeth are common. Of all persons 6 to 50 years of age, 25% had sustained an injury that resulted in damage to one or more anterior teeth.[30] In 1991, more than 5.9 million injuries were treated in dental offices.[55] In 1993 and 1994, 20 million visits to emergency departments were due to craniofacial injuries.[1] Of the 2.9 million emergency department visits in 1997 and 1998 for oral injuries, 25% were reported in children under age 4 years.[1]

Different rates of emergency department visits have been reported among demographic groups. The leading causes of injuries to the head, face, and teeth are falls, assaults, sports-related activities, and bicycle and automobile collisions.[1, 56] Community-based interventions, professional practices, and personal behaviors that increase the use of passenger restraints, air bags, helmets, protective gear, and mouth guards can prevent oral injuries in the future.

Dental Fluorosis

In a 1986–1987 national survey of American schoolchildren, dental fluorosis was present in 22.3% (grades 2–12) examined using Dean's Fluorosis Index.[57] The survey included children exposed to all sources of fluoride. The dental fluorosis by classification was:

- Very mild, 17%
- Mild, 4%
- Moderate, 1%
- Severe, 0.3%

Thus, 77.7% of children were found to not have fluorosis.[57] This study is the only national survey of dental fluorosis, and its results can serve as a baseline for future assessments in the United States.

ACCESS TO THE ORAL HEALTH CARE SYSTEM

Barriers to Dental Care

Many children and adults in the United States do not receive clinical dental care that is essential for their healthy growth, development, and well-being. Americans of all ages can gain improved oral health with increased access to appropriate, timely, and quality dental care. A host of barriers that prevent timely use of personal oral health services have been identified and include barriers related to patients, professionals, the oral health care system, and society. Some key barriers include the following[1]:

- Cost
- Lack of perceived need for regular dental care
- Lack of dental insurance

- ◆ Lack of dental providers
- ◆ Fear of dental visits

Vulnerable population groups, including low-income elderly people, homeless persons, migrant and seasonal farmworkers, disabled and medically compromised individuals, rural residents, and very young children, often lack access to dental care.[58]

Regular Dental Visits and Utilization of Dental Services

The percentage of people in the United States who have had at least one dental visit annually and the average number of visits vary among population groups. Regular dental attendance changes significantly according to age, race and ethnicity, dental status, level of education, and family income.[4] According to the National Health Interview Survey in 1997, 65% of the total United States population over age 2 years had a dental visit in the past year.

Children aged 2 to 4 years are least likely to have had an annual dental visit, whereas a much larger proportion of these children have had well-child visits and have received immunizations, health care, or counseling.[59] It has been reported that only 45% of children in this age group had a dental visit in the past year. According to the 1997 Survey, 11% of children aged 2 to 17 years had a dental visit that was associated with pain in a 1-year period and 20% of poor children had such a visit.[1]

Older people are less likely to schedule dental visits on a regular basis. Of people 65 years of age and older, 54% reported a dental visit. Among dentate adults, 67% had a dental visit in the past year; among edentulous adults, the rate was 37%.[4] Only 19% of nursing home residents had an annual dental visit. One in seven adults reported experiencing dental pain over a 6-month period.[1]

According to NHANES III, 31% of poor adults 18 years and older had a dental visit in the last year, compared with 37% of those with near-poor income and 59% of adults with middle-level or high-level family income.[31] The Medical Expenditures Panel Survey found in 1996 that low-income children experienced the highest disease prevalence, the most extensive disease, the most frequent bouts of dental pain, but the fewest dental visits despite the comprehensive coverage now promised under Medicaid and the new state Children's Health Insurance Program.[60]

Disparities related to regular dental attendance are shown in Tables 4–7 and 4–8.

Unmet Dental Needs

In 1994, 8% of the United States population wanted, but could not obtain, needed dental care.[61] About 16% of individuals from households with low family incomes (e.g., poor and near-poor) reported unmet dental care

Table 4–7

Disparities in Use of the Oral Health Care System (Annual Dental Visit)

Population Groups	Annual Dental Visit (%)*
All (>2 yr old)	65
Race and Ethnicity	
American Indian or Alaska Native†	25
Asian or Pacific Islander	62
African American	57
White	66
Hispanic	53
Education Level (aged 25 yr and older)§	
< High school	41
High school graduate	59
> High school	74
Gender	
Female	67
Male	63
Disability Status	
Persons with disabilities	58
Persons without disabilities	67
Select Populations	
Third grade students	82
Children 2–21 yr, <200% of poverty level	61
Adults 18+ yr	63
Adults 65+ yr	54
Dentate adults 18+ yr	67
Edentate adults 18+ yr	34
Adults 18+ yr with disabilities	52
Long-term care residents‡	19

* National Health Interview Survey, 1997, Centers for Disease Control, National Center for Health Statistics.

† Annual Patient Registration Management System, 1999, Indian Health Service.

‡ National Nursing Home Survey, 1997, Centers for Disease Control and Prevention, National Center for Health Statistics.

§ Level of education (high school) is defined as that of head of household.

Adapted from Centers for Disease Control and Prevention, Healthy People 2000 Review, 1999–2000. Hyattsville, Md, Public Health Service, 1999[31]; and Healthy People 2010: Understanding and Improving Health (Conference ed, 2 vols). Washington, DC, U.S. Department of Health and Human Services, 2000.[4]

Table 4–8
Disparities: Children and Adolescents*
(<19 years, at or Below 200% of Federal Poverty Level)
with Preventive Dental Visit in 1996

Population Groups	Percent (%)
All	20
Race and Ethnicity	
African American	13
White	25
Hispanic	16
Gender	
Female	21
Male	19

Data from National Medical Expediture and Panel Survey, 1996, Agency for Health Care Policy and Research.

Adapted from Centers for Disease Control and Prevention, Healthy People 2000 Review, 1999–2000. Hyattsville, Md, Public Health Service, 1999.[31]

needs.[61] More than 22% of persons who were uninsured reported unmet dental care needs.[61] Among children whose parents reported an unmet health care need, 73% of them had an unmet dental need, according to analysis of the National Health Interview Survey.[62] When communities assess their own health care needs, dental care is frequently cited as a primary unmet need.[2]

Dental Care Coverage

Young and Older Adults

In 1997, more than 95% of dental expenditures were paid by private sources, either out of pocket (47.9%) or by private dental insurance (47.1%).[63] Spending for dental services in the United States has risen steadily but has remained fairly constant as a proportion of personal health care spending (~4.5%).

Dental insurance coverage has not increased; approximately 108 million children and adult Americans have no form of dental insurance.[1] Only 45% of persons in the United States have some form of private dental insurance (most with limited coverage and high co-payments), 9% have public dental insurance (Medicaid and Children's Health Insurance Program), 2% have other dental insurance, and 45% have no dental insurance.[1] A large proportion of adults without dental insurance are between ages 18 and 24 years or over 55 years of age. The out-of-pocket costs for dental care can be a significant burden on low-income Americans.[64, 65]

Often dental care in the private sector is not accessible for many Americans, especially those from vulnerable groups.[64]

Dental care coverage for adults is optional in Medicaid and available in about 60% of the states. Fifteen states provide full coverage for adults, and 18 states provide partial coverage with many limitations. In 18 states, no services or only emergency services are available for adult dental care.[59, 65] Only 15% of older adults have any private dental insurance, and Medicare does not provide reimbursement for routine dental services. Medicare dental benefits are not authorized, with the limited exception of special dental care associated with systemic diseases and their treatment.

Children and Adolescents

According to the National Health Interview Survey in 1995, more than 10 million children lack health insurance and more than 23 million (36% of American children) lack dental insurance. For every child with no medical coverage, there are about 2.6 children in the United States with no dental coverage. Many more children are underinsured for dental care; they may receive an oral examination and prophylaxis but not needed treatment of disease.

All states provide dental care to children under Medicaid and its Early Periodic Screening, Diagnostic, and Treatment (EPSDT) program, according to the Health Care Financing Administration (HCFA).[66] In 1996, 22.9 million children were eligible for this program.[66] Twenty-five percent of children in the United States are covered under EPSDT, which mandates comprehensive dental care.[66] Only 20% of children covered by Medicaid received a preventive dental visit in fiscal year 1993.[59] Of children enrolled in Medicaid, 30% had a dental visit for any reason in fiscal year 1999.[65] Medicaid reports that 80% of children receive regular pediatric care, whereas fewer than 20% receive any preventive dental services.[67] Yet only 2.5% of Medicaid children's health care costs are spent on oral health services.

The state Children's Health Insurance Program (CHIP) provides important new opportunities for improving access to dental care for children from low-income and modest-income families. Dental caries is increasingly a disease of such children—children covered by CHIP. In many instances, dental caries remains untreated.[41] Although dental care is an optional benefit in CHIP, 54 of 56 states and territories include substantial dental services in the approved benefit package for CHIP; two states (Colorado and Delaware) do not include dental care.[67]

Recent studies have shown that cost of dental care in Medicaid is disproportionate for a few, and most often young, preschool-aged children. These studies have found that a small percentage (~2% to 5%) of low-income children with devastating early childhood caries consume an overwhelmingly disproportionate share of Medicaid spending (25% to 45%).[67-69] The cost to Medicaid for treatment of a very young child in the hospital under general anesthesia for restorative dental care was reported as $1500 to $2000 per episode.[68, 69] Treatment of early childhood dental caries, a preventable disease, is expensive when the disease is not prevented, detected, or controlled early. Medicaid spends at least $100 million per year for operating room charges associated with early childhood caries in very young children.[67]

Early primary prevention and greater continuity of dental care for young children at highest risk for dental caries have been emphasized in recent reports.[68, 69] This early intervention (EI) for early childhood caries holds promise for improving health and lowering public expenditures. It has been recognized that long-standing, complex barriers limit the potential of Medicaid to provide needed oral health services to low-income children.[59] It is crucial that oral health programs within Medicaid and CHIP be upgraded and improved continuously to ensure the best outcomes and benefits. Organizations and agencies at the national and state levels have begun to discuss and implement ways to address dental care access problems for children.[1, 70, 71] It is essential that these discussions focusing on children be expanded to ensure access to dental services for all adults in the United States.

▧ ORAL HEALTH CARE SYSTEM

Changing demographics within the United States will have a long-term impact on the oral health care system in the future. These changes will affect patients and providers of oral health care services. Innovative strategies are needed to recruit and retain dental professionals from specific racial and ethnic groups who will seek careers in oral health and public health, today and in the future. With the current oral health care disparities and expected demographic shifts in the population, creative measures are essential for all aspects of oral health, including education, research, health promotion, and clinical care within the private, public, and nonprofit sectors.

Supply and Distribution of Dental Professionals

Most dental care is provided in the private sector; 92% of active dentists in the United States are in private practice and the majority are in solo or two-doctor offices.[72] The employment status for dentists shows that 79% are sole proprietors, 13% are partners, 6% are non-owner dentists, and 2% are independent contractors.[72] The ratio of general dentists to specialists has remained stable at 4 to 1. Owing to changes in public policies, it is projected that this may decrease to 3 to 1.

The ratio of dentists to population increased in the 1980s and decreased in the 1990s as a result of the changing number of dentists entering and leaving the workforce.[73, 74] In 1980, there were an estimated 53.6 dentists per 100,000 persons.[1] This ratio increased to 59.1 per 100,000 people in 1990 and decreased to 58.3 in 2000. By the year 2010, the ratio of dentists to population is expected to decrease to 57.2 and to decline even further, to 53.7 in 2020.[1] In contrast, the ratio of physicians to population has been increasing steadily since 1990.[1, 75]

Dentists in the United States are distributed unevenly and are underrepresented in areas of high need. Dental practices tend to be disproportionately concentrated in suburban areas with high income and education levels, with dentists less available in inner cities or rural areas.[1] Availability of dentists differs markedly among states—the dentist-to-population ratio ranges from 37.2 per 100,000 in Nevada to 78.6 per 100,000 in Connecticut.[74] During the year 2000, 1178 dental health professional shortage areas were designated in the United States.[76]

The number of underrepresented minority dentists is inadequate relative to the rapid growth among racial and ethnic minority groups. African Americans account for 12% of the general population but only 2% of active dentists. Hispanics make up nearly 11% of the population but only 3% of active dentists. Underrepresented minority dentists are more likely to provide care to minority populations. African American dentists report that nearly 62% of their patients are African Americans, and about 45% of the patients of Hispanic dentists are Hispanic.[77] Of the 16,570 undergraduate dental students enrolled in dental schools during 1996 to 1997, representation by racial and ethnic groups was as follows[74]:

- ◆ Asian, 21.8%
- ◆ Black, 5.7%
- ◆ Hispanic, 5.0%
- ◆ Native American, 0.5%
- ◆ White, 67.0%

The greatest gains in dental school enrollment have been in increased representation of females. New female enrollees increased from 5% in 1970 to 38% in 1999.[73]

There are approximately 100,000 dental hygienists, 200,000 dental assistants, and 70,000 dental laboratory technicians in the United States. Figure 4–3 summarizes the current status of students in dental professions.

Public Financing

The proportion of dental care paid for with government revenues is small and declining. In 1997, less than 5% of the estimated $50.64 billion

	Dental	Dental hygiene	Dental assisting	Dental laboratory technology
Schools and programs	54	216	228	34
Total student enrollment	16,570	11,207	7,211	1,141
Graduates	3,930	4,771	4,343	383

Figure 4–3. Summary of students in dental professions (1996–1997). (Data from Trends in Dental Education 2000: The Past, Present, and Future of the Profession or the People It Serves. Washington, D.C., American Association of Dental Schools, January 1999.)

Figure 4–4. Dental public health infrastructure and capacity in the United States. (Adapted from Association of State and Territorial Dental Directors: Building Infrastructure and Capacity in State and Territorial Oral Health Programs, 2000.[80])

• 34 full-time state dental directors and a total of 418 full-time equivalent positions in states
• 473 local health departments with dental programs
• 855 community-based low-income dental clinics
• 290 school-based or school-linked dental programs

spent on dental care was paid by public dollars. That proportion has been declining since the 1960s. Of the $2.27 billion spent on dental care from public funds, $1.12 billion was directed to federal Medicaid, $0.87 billion to state and local Medicaid, and $0.07 billion to Medicare.[63, 78]

Federal, state, and local governments support a wide array of oral health programs that may include direct care services.[79] Figure 4–4 illustrates the dental public health infrastructure and capacity in the United States in 2000. Sources of funding of state programs are varied and include state and federal monies. States are supported by federal funding from two main sources[80]:

◆ Maternal and Child Health Block Grant of the Health Resources and Services Administration (HRSA)
◆ Preventive Health Block Services Grant of the CDC

The infrastructure and personnel capacity of many dental public health programs are limited in comparison with the needs in states and communities.[7]

The publicly funded and "safety net" dental delivery system is under pressure and in short supply.[58] The nation's 3000 federally funded health centers are meeting just 6% of the need for dental care.[81] The distribution of the dental work force is placing stress on the public, nonprofit, and private sectors that provide services in the oral health care system. This is causing reductions in access to oral health services in rural and central city locations.[78, 82]

▨ FUTURE DIRECTIONS

Progress in oral health will be influenced by future trends. Assessments will be important to monitor changes in:

◆ Oral health and disease patterns
◆ Use of services
◆ Social, demographic, and economic factors
◆ Work force and service system capacity (public, private, and non-profit sectors)

The release of *Oral Health in America* by the Surgeon General, the launch of oral health objectives in *Healthy People 2010,* and the progress report for *Healthy People 2000* offer focused attention and a framework for future improvements. They display successes of the 20th century but also outline challenges ahead and propose opportunities to reduce oral health disparities in the 21st century. These reports as well as the publication of the American Dental Association *Future of Dentistry Report* outline options that, when combined with political will can produce oral health improvements for everyone in the United States.

Summary

This chapter has presented the goals and health objectives of *Healthy People 2010;* these benchmarks provide an important framework for the assessment of health in the United States in the coming decade. The chapter has described the clinical and nonclinical measures used in evaluating oral health in populations and the importance of standardizing measurements to assess oral health status and access to oral health services to improve consistency of findings among oral health surveys in communities.

Key oral health indicators in the United States, the current status and past trends of oral health and access to oral health care services, and the determinants of oral health have been explained in the chapter. Also, the chapter presents an overview of behavioral, social, environmental, and economic factors that influence oral health in populations. Finally, important oral health disparities among population groups based on race and ethnicity, family income, education level, gender, geographic location, and disability have been brought to light.

APPLYING YOUR KNOWLEDGE

1. Apply your knowledge about community assessment and oral health surveys.
   a. Select three oral health objectives from *Healthy People 2010.*
   b. For each objective, describe how you would assess it in the coming year in the following situations:
   Objective 1—in an urban inner city community
   Objective 2—in a suburban community
   Objective 3—in a rural county
2. Read over the following situations and questions. Discuss your ideas and answers in small groups.

   a. The chair of the Healthy Communities Task Force contacts you at the State Health Department. The number 1 priority issue for the Task Force is fluoridation of the municipal water supply. The Task Force is interested in your technical assistance in developing this local initiative and would like your suggestions about assessments in the community that are necessary to get this initiative implemented in the coming year. What assessment issues might the Task Force need to address? Whom should they contact? What steps may it need to take? How could this community process instigate the development and implementation of a community oral health improvement plan?

b. ARC, a community-based organization that provides vocational opportunities for disabled adults, has become concerned about its clients' dental status and lack of access to dental care. A legislator from this rural area takes up this issue and is interested in improving access to dental care for adults. She asks her legislative aide to evaluate the dental access problems and to study the options in the Medicaid program to provide dental coverage for low-income adults, especially adults with disabilities. Representatives from a State Disability Coalition meet with you at the State Health Department to discuss your insights. The next day, the Executive Director of the State Association of Community Health Centers calls you and asks you to describe some of the barriers to dental care that adults face in rural counties across the state. How would you capitalize on these unique circumstances to develop a state oral health assessment? Whom would you contact? What steps would you take? How could these activities contribute to the development and implementation of a state oral health improvement plan?

Dental Hygiene Competencies

Reading the material in this chapter and participating in the activities of Applying Your Knowledge will contribute to the student's ability to demonstrate the following competencies:

Health Promotion and Disease Prevention
HP.4 Identify individual and population risk factors and develop strategies that promote health-related quality of life.

Community Involvement
CM.1 Assess the oral health needs of the community and the quality and availability of resources and services.

Patient/Client Care
PC.1 Systematically collect, analyze, and record data on the general, oral, and psychosocial health status of a variety of patients or clients using methods consistent with medicolegal principles.
PC.2 Use critical decision-making skills to reach conclusions about the patient's or client's dental hygiene needs based on all available assessment data.
PC.5a Determine the outcomes of dental hygiene interventions using indices, instruments, examination techniques, and the patient's or client's self-report.

References

1. Oral Health in America: A Report of the Surgeon General. Rockville, Md, U.S. Department of Health and Human Services, National Institute of Dental and Craniofacial Research, National Institutes of Health, 2000.

2. Meyer JA, Silow-Carroll S: Increasing access: Building working solutions from the Kellogg Foundation's Community Voices Initiative. Washington, DC, Economic and Social Research Institute, 2000.

3. Cohen LK, Gift HC (eds): Disease Prevention and Oral Health Promotion: Socio-dental Sciences in Action. Copenhagen, Munksgaard, 1995.

4. Healthy People 2010: Understanding and Improving Health (Conference ed, 2 vols). Washington, DC, U.S. Department of Health and Human Services, 2000.

5. Healthy People 2000: National Health Promotion and Disease Prevention Objectives. Washington, DC, U.S. Department of Health and Human Services, 1990.

6. Healthy People: Surgeon General's Report on Health Promotion and Disease Prevention. Washington, DC, U.S. Department of Health, Education, and Welfare, 1979.

7. Building Infrastructure and Capacity in State and Territorial Oral Health Programs. Association of State and Territorial Dental Directors, 2000.

8. White JA, Beltran ED: Training Manual for Standardized Oral Health Screening, rev ed. Atlanta, Centers for Disease Control and Prevention, 2000.

9. Basic Screening Surveys: An Approach to Monitoring Community Oral Health. Association of State and Territorial Dental Directors, Screening Training Project, 1999.

10. Essential State Dental Public Health Services to Promote Oral Health in the United States: Guidelines for State and Territorial Oral Health Programs. Association of State and Territorial Dental Directors, 1997.

11. Association of State and Territorial Dental Directors (ASTDD): Assessing Oral Health Needs: ASTDD Seven-Step Model. Arlington, Va, National Center for Education in Maternal and Child Health, 1997.

12. Carnahan BW: Oral Health Examination Survey Manual (companion document to Assessing Oral Health Needs: ASTDD Seven-Step Model). Arlington, Va, National Center for Education in Maternal and Child Health, 1997.

13. Vargas C, Schober S, Gift HC: Operational definitions for year 2000 objectives: Priority area 13, oral health. Statistical Notes, No. 12, May 1997.

14. Drury TF, Winn DM, Snowden CB, et al: An overview of the oral health component of the 1988–1991 National Health and Nutrition Examination Survey (NHANES III, Phase 1) (special issue). J Dent Res 75:620, 1996.

15. Oral Health Surveys: Basic Methods, 4th ed. Geneva, World Health Organization, 1997.

16. Burt BA, Eklund SA: Dentistry, Dental Practice, and the Community, 5th ed. Philadelphia, WB Saunders, 1999.

17. Wilkins EM: Clinical Practice of the Dental Hygienist. Philadelphia, Lippincott Williams & Wilkins, 1999.

18. Kaste LM, Selwitz RJ, Oldakowski RJ, et al: Coronal caries in the primary and permanent dentition of children and adolescents 1–17 years of age: United States, 1998–1991 (special Issue). J Dent Res 75:631, 1996.

19. Winn DM, Brunelle JA, Selwitz RJ, et al: Coronal and root caries in the dentition of adults in the United States, 1988–1999 (special issue). J Dent Res 75:642, 1996.

20. White BA, Albertini TF, Brown LJ, et al: Selected restoration and tooth conditions: United States, 1988–1991 (special issue). J Dent Res 75:661, 1996.

21. Lewitt EM, Kerrebrock N: Child indicators: Dental health. Future Child 8:133, 1998.

22. Selwitz RH, Winn DM, Kingman A, Zion GR: The prevalence of dental sealants in the US population: Findings from NHANES III, 1988–1991 (special issue). J Dent Res 75:652, 1996.

23. American Academy of Periodontology: Consensus report on periodontal diseases: Epidemiology and diagnosis. Ann Periodontol 1:216, 1996.

24. Brown LJ, Brunelle JA, Kingman A: Periodontal status in the United States, 1988–1991: Prevalence, extent, and demographic variation (special issue). J Dent Res 75:672, 1996.

25. Drury TF, Brown LJ, Zion GR: Tooth retention and tooth loss in the permanent dentition of adults: United States, 1988–1991 (special issue). J Dent Res 75:684, 1996.

26. Centers for Disease Control and Prevention: National Health Interview Survey 1998 Questionnaire: Adult Prevention Module. Hyattsville, Md, National Center for Health Statistics, Centers for Disease Control and Prevention, June 27, 2000.

27. Brunelle JA, Bhat M, Lipton JA: Prevalence and distribution of selected occlusal characteristics in the U.S. population, 1988–1991 (special issue). J Dent Res 75:706, 1996.

28. Cons NC, Jenny J, Kohout FJ: DAI: The Dental Aesthetic Index. Iowa City, University of Iowa College of Dentistry, 1986.
29. Tolarova MM, Cervenka J: Classification and prevalence of orofacial clefts. Am J Med Genet 75:126, 1998.
30. Kaste LM, Gift HC, Bhat M, Swango PA: Prevalence of incisor trauma in persons 6 to 50 years of age: United States, 1988–1991 (special issue). J Dent Res 75:696, 1996.
31. Centers for Disease Control and Prevention, National Center for Health Statistics: Healthy People 2000 Review, 1999–2000. Hyattsville, Md, Public Health Service, 1999.
32. Warren RC: Oral Health for All: Policy for Available, Accessible, and Acceptable Care. Washington, DC, Center for Policy Alternatives, September 1999.
33. Schou L, Blinkhorn AS: Oral Health Promotion. New York, Oxford University Press, 1993.
34. Weintraub JA: Uses of oral health related quality of life measures in public health. Community Dent Health 15:8, 1998.
35. Slade GD, Strauss RP, Atchison KA, et al: Conference summary: Assessing oral health outcomes—measuring health status and quality of life. Community Dent Health 15:3, 1998.
36. Chen M, Andersen RM, Barmes DE, et al: Comparing Oral Health Care Systems: A Second International Collaborative Study. Geneva, World Health Organization, 1997.
37. Gift HC, Reisine ST, Larch DC: The social impact of dental problems and visits. Am J Public Health 82:1663, 1993.
38. Acs G, Lodolinni G, Kaminski S, et al: Effect of nursing caries on body weight in a pediatric population. J Pediatr Dent 14:302, 1992.
39. Seif A: Promoting Awareness, Preventing Pain: Facts on Early Childhood Caries. Arlington, Va, Maternal and Child Health Bureau, U.S. Department of Health and Human Services and National Maternal and Child Oral Health Resource Center, 1999.
40. Reisine S, Douglas JM: Psychological and behavioral issues in early childhood caries. Community Dent Oral Epidemiol 26:32, 1998.
41. Vargas CM, Crall JJ, Schneider DA: Sociodemographic distribution of pediatric dental caries: NHANES III, 1988–1994. J Am Dent Assoc 129:1229, 1998.
42. Centers for Disease Control and Prevention, National Center for Health Statistics: Healthy People 2000 Review, 1998–1999. Hyattsville, Md, Public Health Service, 1998.
43. Gift HC, Corbin SB, Nowjack-Raymer RE: Public knowledge of prevention of dental disease. Public Health Rep 109:397,1994.
44. Centers for Disease Control and Prevention: Fluoridation of drinking water to prevent dental caries. MMWR Morb Mortal Wkly Rep 48:933, 1999.
45. 1998 Consumers' Opinions Regarding Community Water Fluoridation. Chicago, American Dental Association, 1998.
46. Centers for Disease Control and Prevention: Knowledge of the purpose of community water fluoridation: United States, 1990. MMWR Morb Mortal Wkly Rep 41:919, 1992.
47. Centers for Disease Control and Prevention: Preventing and controlling oral and pharyngeal cancer: Recommendations from a national strategic planning conference. MMWR Morb Mortal Wkly Rep 47(RR14):1, 1998.
48. Cancer facts and figures. Atlanta, American Cancer Society, 1999.
49. Wingo PA, Ries LA, Giovino GA, et al: Annual report to the nation on the status of cancer, 1973–1996. J Natl Cancer Inst 91:675, 1999.
50. Ries LA, Kosary CL, Hankey BF, et al (eds): SEER Cancer Statistics Review, 1973–1996. Bethesda, Md, National Cancer Institute, 1999.
51. Peto R, Lopez A, Boreham J, et al (eds): Tobacco and Health: Proceedings of the 9th World Conference on Tobacco and Health. New York, Plenum Press, 1995.
52. Centers for Disease Control and Prevention, National Center for Health Statistics: Data 2010: The Healthy People 2010 Database (Conference ed), Focus Area 21—Oral Health. Hyattsville, Md, January 2000.
53. Horowitz AM, Nourjah PA, Gift HC: U.S. adult knowledge of risk factors and signs of oral cancers: 1990. J Am Dent Assoc 126:39, 1995.
54. Horowitz AM, Nourjah PA: Factors associated with having oral cancer examinations among U.S. adults 40 years of age and older. J Public Health Dent 56:331, 1996.
55. Gift HC, Bhat M: Dental visits for orofacial injury: Defining the dentist's role. J Am Dent Assoc 124:92,1993.
56. Zeng Y, Sheller B, Milgrom P: Epidemiology of dental emergency visits to a children's hospital. Pediatr Dent 16:419, 1994.
57. U.S. Department of Health and Human Services, Public Health Service (USDHHS, PHS): Review of Fluoride: Benefits and Risks. Report of the Ad Hoc Subcommittee on Fluoride. Washington, DC, USDHHS, PHS, February 1991.

58. U.S. General Accounting Office: Oral Health: Factors Contributing to Low Use of Dental Services by Low-Income Populations. Washington, DC, U.S. General Accounting Office, September 2000.

59. Children's Dental Services under Medicaid: Access and Utilization (No. OE1-09-93-00240). San Francisco, U.S. Department of Health and Human Services, Office of the Inspector General, 1996.

60. Edelstein BL, Manski RJ: Pediatric dental visits during 1996: An analysis of the federal Medical Expenditure Panel Survey. Pediatr Dent 22:17, 2000.

61. Mueller CD, Shur CL, Paramore LC: Access to dental care in the United States. J Dent Educ 129:429, 1998.

62. Newacheck PW, Hughes DC, Hung Y-Y, et al: The unmet health needs of America's children. Pediatrics 105(Suppl):989,2000.

63. Allukian M: Dental Insurance Is Essential But Not Enough. Washington, DC, Closing the Gap, Office of Minority Health, July 1999.

64. Kenney GM, Ko G, Ormond BA: Gaps in Prevention and Treatment: Dental Care for Low-income Children. Washington, DC, The Urban Institute, New Federalism, National Survey of America's Families Series B (No. B-15), April 2000.

65. Dental Disease Is a Chronic Problem Among Low-income Populations. Washington, DC, U.S. General Accounting Office, April 2000.

66. Dental Coverage under Medicaid. Washington, DC, Center for Policy Alternatives, September 1999.

67. Innovative Management of Dental Decay for Young Children Enrolled in Medicaid and CHIP [Children's Health Insurance Program] (grant demonstration program announcement). Baltimore, Health Care Financing Administration, U.S. Department of Health and Human Services, May 2000.

68. Kanellis MJ, Damiano PC, Momany ET: Medicaid costs associated with hospitalization of young children for restorative dental treatment under general anesthesia. J Public Health Dent 60:28, 2000.

69. Griffin SO, Gooch BF, Beltran E, et al: Dental services, costs, and factors associated with hospitalization for Medicaid-eligible children. J Public Health Dent 60:21, 2000.

70. American Dental Association: Proceedings: Report of Achieving Improvement in Medicaid (AIM) for Change Medicaid Conference, August 2–3, 1999.

71. Spisak S, Holt K (eds): Building Partnerships to Improve Children's Access to Medicaid Oral Health Services: National Conference Proceedings. Arlington, Va, National Maternal and Child Oral Health Resource Center, 1999.

72. Distribution of Dentists in the United States by Region and State, 1998. Chicago, American Dental Association, January 2000.

73. Trends in Dental Education 2000: The Past, Present and Future of the Profession or the People It Serves. Washington, DC, American Association of Dental Schools, January 1999.

74. Health Resources and Services Administration: United States Health Workforce Personnel Factbook. Rockville, Md, U.S. Department of Health and Human Services, 2000.

75. Health Resources and Services Administration: United States Health Workforce Personnel Factbook. Rockville, Md, U.S. Department of Health and Human Services, 1997.

76. Health Resources and Services Administration: Health professional shortage area designations. Washington, DC: Federal Register, September 15, 2000.

77. Brown LJ, Lazar V: Minority Dentists: Why Do We Need Them? Washington, DC, Closing the Gap, Office of Minority Health, July 1999.

78. Reports on National Health Care Expenditures. Baltimore, Health Care Financing Administration, Office of the Actuary, 1997.

79. State of the States: Overview of 1999 State Legislation on Access to Oral Health Care. Washington, DC, Center for Policy Alternatives, December 1999.

80. Synopsis of State and Territorial Dental Public Health Programs. Association of State and Territorial Dental Directors, April 2000.

81. Health insurance report: Second-class medicine. Consumer Reports, September 2000, pp 42–50.

82. Barnett WS, Brown KC: Dental Health Policy Series: Issues in Children's Access to Dental Care under Medicaid. Chicago, American Dental Association, April 2000.

Oral Health Programs in the Community

Sherry Jenkins, RDH, BS
Kathy Voigt Geurink, RDH, MA
Linda Altenhoff, DDS

OBJECTIVES

Upon completion of this chapter, the student will be able to:

♦ Identify oral health programs at the national, state, and local level

♦ Discuss the essential public health services for oral health

♦ Describe the four phases of organizing an effective community oral health program

♦ Define goals and objectives

♦ Explain how program goals and objectives are used in program planning, implementation, and evaluation

♦ Discuss the benefits of primary prevention programs, including fluoridation, sealants, and oral health education

♦ Describe the importance of community water fluoridation as a public health measure

♦ Identify the different funding streams and structures for obtaining dental services through public health systems

Essential Public Health
    Services for Oral Health

Oral Health Coalition

Assessment

Planning

Implementation

Evaluation

Goals

Objectives

Community Water
    Fluoridation

Sealants

Oral Health Education

Opening Statement

Community Oral Health Programs

◆ *Community Dental Sealant Programs*

◆ *Tobacco Cessation and Spit Tobacco Programs*

◆ *Water Fluoridation Programs*

◆ *Oral Health Coalitions*

◆ *Early Childhood Caries Programs*

◆ *Geriatric Dental Programs*

◆ *School Fluoride Mouth Rinse Programs*

◆ *Needs Assessment and Oral Health Surveys*

▨ GENERAL HEALTH AND ORAL HEALTH

The mission of public health is to "fulfill society's interest in assuring conditions in which people can be healthy."[1] Without public health, including community oral health, society as a whole suffers because of lost productivity, decreased learning among our school-aged children as a result of health-related absences, and increased health care costs. Surgeon General David Thatcher, in the May 2000 Surgeon General's Report,[2] refers to dental disease as a "silent epidemic that restricts activities in school, work, and home, and often significantly diminishes the quality of life." He further states:

> *To improve the quality of life and eliminate health disparities demands the understanding, compassion, and will of the American people. There are opportunities for all health professionals and communities to work together to improve health.*[2]

This chapter discusses community oral health programs as opportunities for achieving improved oral health and, consequently, overall health.

NATIONAL, STATE, AND LOCAL PROGRAMS: ROLE OF THE HEALTH DEPARTMENT

National Level

National, state, and local dental public health programs have similar roles but widely varying organizational schemes. Nationally, several governmental programs are involved in oral health promotion.

Among these programs are the U.S. Department of Health and Human Services (DHHS), the federal government's principal agency for protecting the health of all Americans and providing essential services, especially for people who are least able to help themselves. DHHS is the largest grant-making agency in the federal government (~60,000 grants per year). DHHS works with state and local governments and funds services at the local level through state or county agencies or through private sector grantees. DHHS also provides regulatory oversight and monitoring of the expenditures made by grantees. DHHS has multiple public health service operating divisions, including:

- National Institutes of Health (NIH)
- Food and Drug Administration (FDA)
- Centers for Disease Control and Prevention (CDC)
- Indian Health Service (IHS)
- Health Resources and Services Administration (HRSA)

State Level

Approximately two thirds of the states have full-time state dental directors who provide leadership and guidance in the planning, funding, and implementation of oral health promotion programs for the residents of the states that they serve. These programs vary in their scope of services and organization across the United States.

A state's program may include, in addition to the state dental director, regional dental directors, public health educators, clinical dentists, dental hygienists, and dental assistants who provide oral health services to underserved populations. These public professionals also promote oral health through educational programs in public and private schools as well as through collaborative efforts with dental and dental hygiene schools; Head Start centers; Women, Infant, and Children (WIC) programs; county and city health departments; community based organizations; faith-based organizations, civic groups; and local dental providers and dental hygienists.

Private practice dental hygienists, through collaboration with state-sponsored oral health promotions, can serve in the roles of Educator/Health Promoter and Consumer Advocate in addition to their role as Clinician, therefore positively affecting the oral health of a greater population base.

Local Level

Individual county and city health departments across the nation have recognized the need within their communities for the provision of oral health services to various members of their populations. Many of these clinics are federally funded, offering services on a sliding scale fee schedule as well as accepting clients who receive public assistance through Medicaid. These clinics employ both public health dentists and dental hygienists and sometimes have supplemental clinical coverage provided by local dental professionals.

Hours of operation are also tailored to best meet the needs of the population that they serve. The clinics provide diagnostic, preventive, and restorative oral health services to the older adults as well as to the indigent population and the working poor.

Essential Public Health Services for Oral Health

The core public health functions of assessment, policy development, and assurance shape the basic practice of public health at state and local levels. These core public health functions and the essential public health services (see Chapter 1) provided input into the **Essential Public Health Services for Oral Health** developed by the Association of State and Territorial Dental Directors (ASTDD) (Fig. 5–1).[3] These guidelines describe the roles of state oral health programs and have been used in the development and evaluation of public health activities at the state level.

Many states have developed programs that include the essential services for oral health. For example, in the State of Washington the *Smile Survey* was initiated to provide statewide screenings for children to assess the status of their oral health and to identify problems. Preventive programs, such as sealants and oral health education, have followed as an answer to the problem of tooth decay. In addition, the Washington State Oral Health Coalition was formed in 1993. A *coalition* is a diverse group of individuals, organizations, and agencies that unite to reach a common goal. An **oral health coalition** is therefore a cooperative effort on the part of many individuals and organizations to build systems and develop programs that improve community oral health.

The Washington State Oral Health Coalition has proved to be an excellent means of bringing dedicated professionals together to resolve oral health issues through policy development. This coalition is also involved in continual assessment of oral health and in the assurance of oral health solutions. More than 20 different locations in Washington have established oral health coalitions, with representation from consumers, schools, community clinics, health care and dental providers, health departments, and agencies that come in contact with low-income and minority populations. Anyone interested in achieving the goal of optimal oral health for

ASSESSMENT
- Assess oral health status and needs so that problems can be identified and addressed
- Analyze determinants of identified oral health needs, including resources
- Assess the fluoridation status of water systems and other sources of fluoride
- Implement an oral health surveillance system to identify, investigate, and monitor oral health problems and health hazards

POLICY DEVELOPMENT
- Develop plans and policies through a collaborative process that supports individual and community oral health efforts to address oral health needs
- Provide leadership to address oral health problems by maintaining a strong oral health unit within the health agency
- Mobilize community partnerships between and among policymakers, professionals, organizations, groups, the public, and others to identify and implement solutions to oral health problems

ASSURANCE
- Inform, educate, and empower the public regarding oral health problems and solutions
- Promote and enforce laws and regulations that protect and improve oral health, ensure safety, and ensure accountability for the public's well-being
- Link people to needed population-based oral health services, personal oral health services, and support services, and assure the availability, access, and acceptability of these services by enhancing system capacity, including directly supporting or providing services when necessary
- Support services and implementation of programs that focus on primary and secondary prevention
- Assure that the public health and personal health work force has the capacity and expertise to effectively address oral health needs
- Evaluate effectiveness, accessibility, and quality of population-based and personal oral health services

Figure 5–1. Essential public health services for oral health. (Adapted from Association of State and Territorial Dental Directors: Guidelines for State and Territorial Oral Health Programs, 1997.[2])

- Provide public recognition and visibility

- Leverage resources; expand the scope and range of services

- Provide a comprehensive approach to programming

- Enhance clout in advocacy and resource development

- Enhance competence

- Avoid duplication of services, and fill gaps in service delivery

- Accomplish what single members cannot

Figure 5–2. Oral health coalitions. (Adapted from Children's Alliance: Washington State Oral Health Coalition. (Available from *http://www.childrensalliance.org/teeth/coalition.htm*.[4])

Washington residents is invited to join. The strength and unity of a coalition make this goal attainable. The Washington Department of Health and the U.S. DHHS have developed a document, *Community Roots for Oral Health: Guidelines for Successful Coalitions,* available to people interested in forming an oral health coalition to improve the oral health of residents in their community (Fig. 5–2).[4]

▨ ASSESSMENT, PLANNING, IMPLEMENTION, AND EVALUATION

Four components are necessary in initiating an oral health program: **assessment, planning, implementation,** and **evaluation** Dental hygienists in private practice and in the community utilize these components to deliver oral health care. Community health extends the role of the dental hygienist from the traditional private practice to the community as a whole.

In this setting, the community is viewed as the patient. The community survey is comparable to the patient's examination for assessment. The program plan and implementation are similar to the treatment plan and treatment of the patient. Evaluation and review of the program can be compared to the evaluation of the patient's treatment (Fig. 5–3).

With increased emphasis on improving public access to oral health care, the responsibilities of the dental hygienist to promote oral health in the community take on renewed importance. Therefore, it is important that the dental hygienist understand the basic concepts of assessment, planning, implementation, and evaluation as they apply to oral health programs.

Definitions of the components of initiating an oral health program follow[5]:

1. *Assessment* is an organized and systematic approach to identify a target group and to define the extent and severity of oral health needs present.

Community		Private Practice
Community survey	← ASSESSMENT →	Patient exam
Plan the program	← PLANNING →	Plan patient treatment
Conduct the program	← IMPLEMENTATION →	Treat the patient
Review program/ evaluate	← EVALUATION →	Evaluate patient treatment

Figure 5–3. Components necessary for initiating an oral health program.

2. *Planning* is an organized response to reduce or eliminate one or more problems.
3. *Implementation* includes the process of putting the plan into action and monitoring the plan's activities, personnel, equipment, resources, and supplies. This step should include feedback from personnel and participants as well as ongoing evaluation mechanisms.
4. *Evaluation* is the method of measuring results of the program against objectives developed during the early planning stages. This process is ongoing and should identify problems and solutions to assist in revising the program as needed.
   a. *Formative evaluation,* or the internal evaluation of a program, is an examination of the processes or activities of a program as they are taking place.
   b. *Summative evaluation* involves judging the merit or worth of a program after it has been in operation. This step is an attempt to determine whether a fully operational program is meeting the goals for which it was developed.

Assessment

Assessing the relative importance of needs can be a complex process. It depends on human values, some of which are universally agreed upon and others that are more controversial. For example, a need that involves life or death generally receives higher priority; however, a choice between a health need that might affect the lives of a few people and one that affects the lives of large numbers of people is less clear-cut. Although many would argue that the needs of larger numbers must take priority, others want to consider factors such as age and the future impact on society. For example, a community may need to decide about initiating a free influenza vaccine program for its older population, enhancing the immunization program for children, or adding a clinic offering reduced dental care for indigent families (see "Guiding Principles," page 138).

Guiding Principles

Establishing Health Priorities

- ◆ What is the magnitude of the problem? (Does it cause death or disability?)

- ◆ How many people are affected (one person, small community, whole country)?

- ◆ What types of resources are available (personnel, money, facilities, technology)?

- ◆ What has already been done in the community?

- ◆ What are the prevailing attitudes toward the problem?

- ◆ Which groups are expressing the most interest in the problem?

- ◆ What are the legal constraints?

Compounding the problem of establishing the priorities of health needs is the fact that each community is unique, with its own values and ideas. If a community's basic need for food and security are not being met, dental needs assume a low priority. An issue that often arises is the idea that if a community's perception of needs is adhered to exclusively, actual clinical health problems may go untreated because the people are not knowledgeable about many areas of health care. The solution to this dilemma involves striking a delicate balance between negligence and overzealousness. Although it is unethical to impose one's own perceptions on a community, it is the professional's responsibility to inform people of existing problems and their consequences.[6]

A needs assessment can identify the problem. The assessment provides information not only about the problem but also about the community itself. The data collected can be used to develop a community profile that will assist in finding the appropriate solution. Conducting a needs assessment for a community can be expensive with regard to labor and time. If funds are not available, coordination with other agencies interested in obtaining similar health information on the given population may be the solution.

Another possibility is to investigate dental surveys that have been done by other organizations. Dental surveys are conducted by professionals at dental schools, local and state health departments, and community health centers. Coordination with other agencies and organizations to know what has been done and what needs to be accomplished can prevent duplication of services.[7] Data can be obtained and analyzed by various methods (see Chapter 3). After the needs assessment, developing the appropriate goals and objectives is the next step.

Planning

Developing goals, objectives, and program activities are part of the planning process. During this stage, it is essential to have community involvement and participation. The formulation of program goals and objectives is an active process, offering specific proposals for changes to be made in the community. These changes address the specific problems identified in the needs assessment.

Goals

Goals provide a broadly based statement of what changes will take place, from which specific objectives are developed, for example: The school-based fluoride mouth rinse program will improve the oral health of school-aged children.

Objectives

Objectives are more specific than goals; they describe, in a measurable way, the desired end result of program activities. They should tell the learner what he or she needs to do to be successful.

The *performance verb* is the key to a measurable objective (Fig. 5–4); it is an action word, such as "write," "demonstrate," or "recite." Other elements of the objective are the *condition*, which tells under what circumstance the activity occurs, and the *criterion*, which tells how well the activity must be performed. The performance verb is essential in writing a measurable objective. The inclusion of a condition and a criterion makes the objective more specific and useful to the learner. In summary:

1. A *performance verb* tells the activity and outcome.
2. A *condition* tells under what circumstance the outcome will occur.
3. A *criterion* tells how well the action and outcome must be accomplished to be effective.

An example of an objective for the aforementioned goal would be as follows: Upon completion of today's six-step demonstration of how to rinse, the children will demonstrate the six steps without error.

Performance verb: demonstrate
Condition: upon completion of today's six-step demonstration
Criterion: without error

Another example of a measurable objective: Upon completion of the calibration exercise, the three examiners will record their findings with an 85% accuracy.

Performance verb: record

Analyze	Examine	Map	State
Apply	Estimate	Measure	Sort
Attempt	Explain	Observe	Spell
Adjust	Express	Organize	Try
Brush	Find	Perform	Test
Calculate	Form	Practice	Unite
Categorize	Gather	Predict	Weigh
Choose	Group	Plan	Write
Classify	Hypothesize	Produce	
Complete	Identify	Prove	
Create	Invent	Record	
Copy	Join	Recognize	
Describe	Keep	Repeat	
Define	Label	Select	
Design	List	Show	
Demonstrate			

Figure 5–4. Performance verbs for writing behavioral objectives.

Condition: Upon completion of the calibration exercise
Criterion: 85% accuracy

Once the problem has been identified and program goals and objectives have been established with a description of a solution, the next step is to state how to bring about the desired results. This area of program planning, referred to as *program activities*, describes how the objectives will be accomplished.

In planning these program activities, one must carefully consider the type of *resources* available as well as program *constraints*. For example, in planning a school fluoride mouth rinse program in which the chosen activity would be weekly rinsing, resources might include selecting (1) the site at which the rinsing is conducted, (2) personnel, (3) supplies, and (4) the financial means to pay for the supplies. Constraints might include (1) availability of dental personnel to conduct screenings, (2) negative attitudes from some parents, (3) the amount of time it takes to rinse, or (4) lack of funding.

Planning is a crucial element to a successful program. A community oral health program that is well planned, with specific activities and consideration to resources and constraints, is usually successful in terms of implementation.

Implementation

The process of putting the plan into action, the implementation phase, is ongoing and should be supervised and evaluated to ensure program effectiveness. Implementation, like planning, involves individuals, agencies, and the community working together. The strategy should answer the following questions[7]:

1. Why: the effect of the objective to be achieved
2. What: the activities required to achieve the objective
3. Who: the individuals responsible for each activity
4. When: the chronologic sequence of activities
5. How: the materials, media, methods, and techniques to be used
6. How much: a cost estimate of materials and time

For ease in addressing these questions, many community oral health programs begin on a small scale. Using a smaller population with the intent to expand later is called *pilot testing*. In a pilot test for a fluoride mouth rinse program, for instance, only one school would be involved the first year and the program would be expanded to include two or more schools the following year. This implementation strategy allows for an opportunity to test the program's effectiveness and provides ease in control and monitoring of the program activities. A pilot program provides useful information and enables decisions to be made about the future of the program. Piloting is a form of evaluating the implementation.

Evaluation

Evaluation is a judgment of merit or worth about the program. The first step is to review the program goals and then to examine the specific measurable objectives. Each objective should be reviewed to determine how well it is meeting the program goals. The bottom line in evaluation is accountability—to consumers, providers, and all involved agencies. Evaluation determines whether the program accomplishes what it was designed to accomplish (e.g., were the objectives of this study or program successfully met? If not, why not?). Summarizing what went well and what did not, or drawing conclusions based on intuition, is not adequate; the objectives themselves must be specifically addressed.

Inherent in this approach is the possibility of attaining a negative outcome, that is, the conclusion that the objectives have not been met. At the same time, however, this does not mean that the program has been a failure. If a program is evaluated properly so that negative outcomes become learning experiences and indicators of future programming and research, in some sense it has been a success.[6] Formative evaluation during the implementation process can point out problems and identify opportunities to correct program deficiencies early on. With ongoing evaluation and change, the summative evaluation (end result) may in fact measure a program with initial problems as successful.

Program evaluation is an example of *applied research*. *Basic (clinical) research* (see Chapter 6) involves inquiry into the truth about facts, behaviors, relationships, and principles. Applied research is concerned with these same concepts but emphasizes the application of the knowledge and developing solutions to problems. For example, a basic researcher would be concerned with the effectiveness of the fluoride mouth rinse on the teeth and which concentration to use. A program evaluator would be concerned with the effect of the program operation and its ability to meet the program objectives. The fundamental purpose of program evaluation is to assist in decision making on the effectiveness of the program in its entirety.

Dental hygienists play a role in assessing, planning, implementing, and evaluating community oral health programs. The dental hygienists who have chosen careers as state dental directors, public health educators, or promoters have played an important role in the advancement of dental public health, but there is much more that can be accomplished by all of the dental hygiene profession. By knowing how to organize an effective community oral health program and becoming involved in its implementation, dental hygienists can have an impact in reaching the goal of optimal oral health care for all people.

▨ PRIMARY PREVENTION PROGRAMS: FLUORIDATION, SEALANTS, ORAL HEALTH EDUCATION

Community Water Fluoridation

Community water fluoridation is the addition of a controlled amount of fluoride to the public water supply with the intent to prevent dental caries in the population. Fluoridation has been recognized as one of the major public health measures of the 20th century:

> *At the turn of the century most Americans could expect to lose their teeth by middle age. That situation began to change with the discovery of the properties of fluoride and the observation that people who lived in communities with naturally fluoridated drinking water had far less dental caries than people in comparable communities without fluoride in their water supply.*[2]

In the 1920s, Dr. Frederick McKay first noticed that people living in regions of Colorado had brown stain on their teeth (*fluorosis*, or mottled enamel) but few, if any, caries. In the 1930s, Dr. Trendley Dean conducted epidemiologic studies to prove the relationship of dental fluorosis, concentration of fluoride in the water, and reduction of dental caries.

Fluoride is the 13th most abundant natural element; it is found in rocks, soil, fresh water, and ocean water. Therefore, trace amounts of fluoride are found in all natural water sources. As a result of the general availability of public water sources to most people, the adjustment of the natural fluoride content found in the water to levels optimal for combating oral disease has proved to be a successful public health measure. This approach provides fluoride to the population, with minimal regard to socioeconomic factors, in a passive vehicle for the consumer. Water fluoridation, accomplished in this manner, results in improved oral health, reduced expenditures for dental restorative procedures, and decreased absences from school and work due to oral pain, with a resultant increase in learning and productivity.

The first city in the United States to adjust the fluoride content in the community water supply was Grand Rapids, Michigan, in the 1940s. Subsequent studies of adjusted fluoridation demonstrated that 50% to 70% of caries were prevented in the permanent teeth of children. Today, decay reduction rates in fluoridated communities are approximately 8% to 37% for children, and 20% to 40% for adults.[8]

Figure 5–5 correlates the percentage of the population residing in areas with fluoridated community water systems and the mean number of decayed, missing (because of caries), or filled permanent teeth (DMFT) among children aged 12 years in the United States from 1967 to 1992. The average number of DMFT steadily declined from 1967 to 1992 because of populations residing in fluoridated communities.[9]

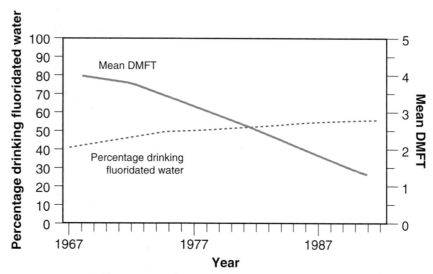

Figure 5–5. Percentage of population residing in areas with fluoridated water systems and with decayed, missing, or filled permanent teeth (DMFT) among children aged 12 years, 1967 to 1992. (Data from Centers for Disease Control and Prevention [CDC]: Fluoridation Census, 1993; CDC, Third National Health and Nutrition Examination Survey, 1988 to 1994; National Center for Health Statistics, 1974 and 1981; and National Institute of Dental Research, 1989.)

Fluoridated Communities

Close to 145 million United States residents benefit from water fluoridation. Of the total population served by public water systems, 62% receive optimally fluoridated water. Figure 5–6 shows the proportion of people on public water systems served by fluoridation in 1992. Figure 5–7 depicts the 50 largest cities and their fluoridation status. The *Healthy People 2010* objective for community water fluoridation is an increase in the proportion of community water systems optimally fluoridated; the target is 75% of the population.[10]

In the United States, fluoridated water is now provided in approximately 10,500 communities, with 14,300 fluoridated community water systems serving the communities. Military bases within the United States as well as in foreign countries have traditionally embraced the public health benefits of water fluoridation by adjusting the fluoride in the base water supply to optimal levels. Figure 5–8 shows the status of water fluoridation in the United States.[10]

Cost of Water Fluoridation

It has been calculated that the mean annual per capita cost of community water fluoridation ranges from $0.68 for systems with a population over 50,000

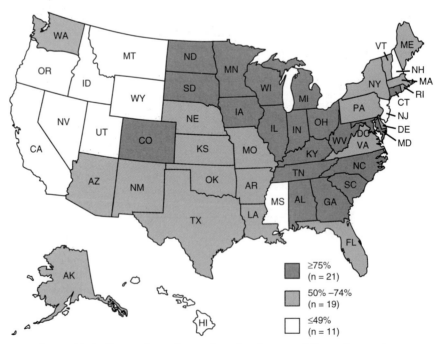

Figure 5–6. Proportion of people who have public water systems served by fluoridation in 1992. (From Centers for Disease Control Fluoridation Census. Atlanta, 1993.)

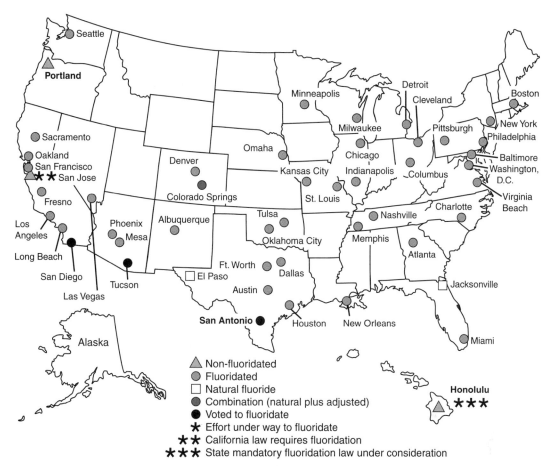

Figure 5–7. Fluoridation status of the 50 largest cities in the United States. (From Centers for Disease Control, 2000, U.S. Census Bureau. Courtesy of University of Texas Health Science Center at San Antonio.)

and $0.98 for systems with a population base between 10,000 and 50,000 to $3.00 for systems with fewer than 10,000 people.[10] The lifetime cost of fluoridation per person is less than the cost of one dental filling. With the escalating cost of health care, fluoridation remains a preventive measure of minimal cost. In determining the economic importance of fluoridation, we should remember that the cost of treating dental disease is paid not only by the affected individual but also by the public through health departments, health insurance premiums, and federally supported programs such as Medicaid.

Optimal Amounts of Fluoride

Several states have fluoridation projects that assist communities in their efforts to assess the need for fluoridation as well as to design and implement fluoridation of their public water systems. The state fluoridation

Status of water fluoridation in the United States as of 12/31/92:

1. **Total U.S. population** 258,544,000
   U.S. population on public water system 232,438,000
   U.S. population NOT on public water system 26,106,000

2. **Total no. of public water supply systems** 59,158
   No. of systems with population less than 100 18,273
   No. of systems with population between 101–500 18,238
   No. of systems with population between 501–1000.... 6,307
   No. of systems with population over 1,000 15,487

3. **Total no. of public water supply systems that are**
   fluoridated 14,351
   Adjusted 10,567
   Natural 3,784

4. **Total no. of fluoridated communities** 10,496
   Adjusted 8,572
   Natural 1,924

5. **Total U.S. population on fluoride drinking**
   water systems .... **144.6 million**
   Adjusted .... 134.6 million
   Natural .... 10.0 million

6. **% of U.S. population receiving fluoridated water .. 55.9%**

7. **% of total U.S. population on public water supply**
   system receiving fluoridated water **62.2%**

Figure 5–8. Fluoridation facts. (Modified from *http://www.cdc.gov/nccdphp/ch/flfact.htm.*)

staff also provides training and technical assistance for local water facility operators.

When the water supply is being fluoridated in a community, climatic temperature and consumption of water are taken into consideration. The recommended levels for water fluoridation in the United States range from 0.7 to 1.2 parts per million (ppm) of fluoride, depending on the average daily temperature for that area. This range is based on the hypothesis that water consumption increases with increasing climatic temperature. This assumption may not be as accurate as earlier research indicates because of the increased use of air conditioning, as well as the increased consumption of soft drinks and bottled water.[11]

Examples of Community Water Fluoridation Programs

INDIANA

An example of a state that has successfully adopted fluoride into its community water systems is Indiana. The Indiana State Department of Health has given community water fluoridation a high priority and had reached the *Healthy People 2010* objective of 75% fluoridation in the 1970s.[12] Grant monies were applied for and secured from departments within the U.S. Public Health Services. As a result of the efforts of dedicated professionals, including dental hygienists fulfilling the roles of Educators, Consumer Advocates, and Change Agents, the state is 98% fluoridated.

The successful implementation of this program can be attributed to effective planning, implementation, and evaluation procedures. In the planning stage, assessment of the community needs and feasibility studies were conducted. The cooperative efforts of professionals, city officials, and citizens result in positive voluntary voting for the implementation of fluoride. Important evaluation measures of the program are the surveillance visits to monitor the amount of fluoride levels in the community drinking water.

More than 1500 surveillance visits are conducted per year to ensure that optimal fluoride levels are maintained. Because of this monitoring, 98% of the 262 fluoridating Indiana communities and 92% of the 56 fluoridating Indiana schools routinely have optimal fluoride levels. Ongoing DMFS surveys convey the successful results of reduced dental decay.[12]

CALIFORNIA

Another state that illustrates a successful effect of a unified effort to implement fluoridation is California. The California Task Force was developed in 1993 and consisted of members from organizations such as the California Dental Association, the California Department of Health, the California Dental Hygiene Association, the California Public Health Association, and the California Dental Health Foundation. The task force created a plan to implement fluoridation in the entire state. Whereas only 17% of California was fluoridated in 1993, today more than 35% of the communities are fluoridated.[13]

For further information on these programs and other state coalitions and task force plans, see the Web sites at the end of this chapter.

Other Fluoride Programs

MOUTH RINSE PROGRAMS

In communities where a public water source is not available or where water fluoridation is undesired for various reasons, school-based fluoride mouth rinse programs have been implemented and offer the benefits of fluoride in a structured environment. Such programs are a popular and cost-effective means of providing fluoride benefits for children. Participation by children in a school-based program requires parental permission and oversight by a licensed dentist.

The mouth rinse program is administered by school personnel or volunteers on a weekly basis to participating children. The children rinse for 60 seconds with 10 ml of 2% sodium fluoride. The fluoride rinse is then expectorated into a paper cup, a napkin is placed inside the cup to absorb the solution, and the cup is discarded. The procedure takes less than 5 minutes.

SCHOOL WATER SUPPLY

Another means of providing fluoridation for schoolchildren in nonfluoridated communities is adding fluoride to the school water system. The amount of fluoride added to the school water is 4.5 times the optimal amount that would be added to the community water. This method is not as readily selected because the amount of water consumed cannot be easily monitored. Limited evidence of effectiveness and difficulties with implementation and operation have led schools to seek alternative preventive methods.

DIETARY FLUORIDE SUPPLEMENTS

The use of dietary fluoride supplements is another popular way of providing fluoride to children. These supplements are available only by prescription and are intended for use by children living in nonfluoridated areas to increase their fluoride exposure to a level equivalent to children who live in optimally fluoridated areas.

Supplements are available in two forms: (1) drops for infants aged 6 months and older and (2) chewable tablets for children and adolescents. To decrease the risk of dental fluorosis in permanent teeth, fluoride supplements should be prescribed only for children living in nonfluoridated areas. The need for continuation of fluoride supplements should be reevaluated in the event of a child's change of residence.

The correct dosage is based on the child's age as well as the existing fluoride level in available drinking water sources (Table 5–1).[14] The water sources to be considered should include:

- Water in the home
- Bottled water
- Water at a school or a day care center
- After-school care sources

The child's risk of decay and all other sources of fluoride exposure, such as through fluoridated toothpastes and food sources, must also be taken into account.

	Table 5–1 Dietary Fluoride Supplement Schedule, 1994*		
Age	**Fluoride Ion Level in Drinking Water (ppm†)**		
	<0.3 ppm	**0.3–0.6 ppm**	**>0.6 ppm**
Birth–6 mo	None	None	None
6 mo–3 yr	0.25 mg/day‡	None	None
3–6 yr	0.50 mg/day	0.25 mg/day	None
6–16 yr	1.0 mg/day	0.50 mg/day	None

* Approved by the American Dental Association, American Academy of Pediatrics, and American Academy of Pediatric Dentistry.

† 1.0 part per million (ppm) = 1 milligram/liter (mg/L)

‡ 2.2 mg of sodium fluoride contains 1 mg of fluoride ion.

Copyright © 2001 American Dental Association. Available from *http://www.ADA.org.*

The need for compliance over an extended period of time is a major procedural and economic disadvantage of community-based fluoride supplement programs. This liability makes them impractical as an alternative to water fluoridation as a public health measure. Although total costs of the purchase of supplements and administration of a program are small, compared with the installation and startup costs associated with fluoridation equipment, the overall cost of supplements per child is much greater than the per capita cost of community water fluoridation. Additionally, community water fluoridation provides decay prevention and oral health benefits for the entire population regardless of age, socioeconomic status, educational attainment, or other social variables. This is particularly important for families and individuals who do not or cannot access regular oral health services.

FLUORIDE VARNISHES

Developed in Europe during the 1960s, fluoride varnishes were introduced into the United States in 1994 and remain in wide use within Europe and Canada. The varnish is applied by an operator, with a recommended twice-yearly reapplication for optimal benefit. The varnish is not intended to be permanent, like a sealant, but to hold the fluoride in contact with the tooth for a period of time. Duraflor, approved by the FDA, has gained popularity in the United States.

Varnishes may be used to prevent root surface caries on adults with gingival recession. They offer easy applicability of fluoride for disabled children or hospitalized patients.[15] Studies in Europe have demonstrated their efficacy.[16] Whether varnishes should be the choice of clinical programs in communities with high caries rates or whether they are better for patients on an individual basis, as needed, has not been determined.

Additional Fluoride Sources

The introduction of *systemic* fluoride through water, vitamins, and tablets during the enamel formation phase of both primary and permanent teeth of children, in utero as well as post partum, provides for optimal dental decay preventive benefits through fluoride ion exchange and resultant denser enamel matrix. Fluoride is provided *topically* through toothpaste, mouth rinses, and professionally prescribed fluoride gels, pastes, rinses, and varnishes. The benefits associated with topical fluoride include the remineralization of early incipient lesions. The effectiveness of various fluoride sources in the reduction of dental caries is shown in Figure 5–9.[17]

With all the additional sources of fluoride available today, the prevalence of caries has decreased but the prevalence of dental fluorosis has increased in both fluoridated and nonfluoridated communities. Factors associated with increased fluorosis today are[17]:

- Early use of fluoride toothpaste
- Use and misuse of dietary supplements
- Consumption of infant formula containing fluoride

Health care professionals, such as dentists, dental hygienists, and physicians, are important sources of information for patients regarding the use of fluoride-containing products, such as toothpaste, and may be able to help reduce the prevalence of enamel fluorosis by educating the public on the appropriate use of these products.

Even though other sources of fluoride are available and despite the increased risk of fluorosis, community water fluoridation remains the most cost-effective, the most practical, and the safest means of preventing tooth decay.

- **Community water fluoridation:** Early studies: 50%–70% reduction in caries, presently 20%–40% reduction in caries due to additional availability of other fluoride sources

- **Mouth rinses:** Studies in the 1970s and 1980s demonstrated a reduction in caries ranging from 20%–50%

- **Fluoride tablet supplements:** Controlled trials in the United States in the 1970s indicated approximately a 20%–28% reduction

- **Toothpaste:** In clinical trials done between 1945 and 1985, 23%–32% reduction in caries

---

Figure 5–9. Community water fluoridation, early studies: 50% to 70% reduction in caries, presently 8% to 37% in children and 20% to 40% in adults. (Data from Milgram P, Reisine S: Oral health in the United States: The post-fluoride generation. Annu Rev Public Health 21:403–406, 2000.)

Antifluoridationists

Antifluoridationists are opponents of community water fluoridation. Their reasons include individual rights, safety, government mistrust, and religious freedom. The arguments against fluoridation do not have any merit based on scientific knowledge. The economic and health benefits of fluoridation for millions of Americans have been confirmed in numerous studies by renowned scientists.[15, 18]

Antifluoridationists attempt to appeal to people's emotions. They provide inaccurate, false information to the public and to the elected officials and attempt to link adverse health effects with fluoridation. Dental hygienists, in the roles of educators and resource persons, can influence the public knowledge about the benefits of fluoridation in their community and can provide scientific, accurate information to the community officials.

For antifluoridationists to be defeated, community education must be executed in a well-planned, unified manner. As active members of the American Dental Hygienists Association and the local components, dental hygienists become an effective force that can have an impact on the community. An organized plan of action can make a difference. Being aware of the issues and being well versed on fluoridation studies and cognizant of the political process are necessary steps in winning a fluoridation campaign. Dental hygienists also work as *Change Agents* in promoting the legislative approval of fluoridation.

Some states and cities have taken administrative action to implement fluoridation; this means that state legislatures and the city council or commission, because of the public health benefits, have voted for fluoridation. People usually prefer to have a voice in the decision-making process; however, if fluoride is on the ballot, people need to be educated on the issue to make a wise decision. Education is the key to the success in reaching the *Healthy People 2010* goal of fluoridation for 75% of the population in the United States.

Dental Sealants

An effective primary preventive strategy, commonly used to protect permanent molars from decay, is the application of **dental sealants.** Although the percentage of school-aged children with sealants has risen in recent years as the public and private sectors have been using the procedure, as dental insurance has paid for the sealants, and as parents have requested sealants for their children, no increase in use has occurred among children in low-income populations. One goal of *Healthy People 2010* is to have 50% of children receiving dental sealants on their permanent molars. According to the 1988–1994 baseline data, only 23% of 8-year-old children and 15% of 14-year-old adolescents had dental sealants on their permanent molars.[19]

To help reach the goal of 50% of children having dental sealants, many states have instituted school-based dental sealant programs. In some programs, mobile dental vans are sent to schools and the sealants are applied in the van. In other programs, portable equipment is transported from school to school and is set up in available spaces. Students are then brought to the designated room for the procedure.

Sealant programs generally focus on 6- to 8-year-olds and 12- to 14-year-olds because the first and second molars usually erupt during these years. Placing sealants on these teeth shortly after their eruption protects them from development of caries in areas where food and bacteria are retained. If sealants were applied routinely to susceptible tooth surfaces in conjunction with the appropriate use of fluoride, most tooth decay in children could be prevented.

The "Seal a Smile" program in Wisconsin is an example of a primary prevention program to promote dental sealants to all children who need them. Funded by a grant from the CDC, the program is part of an initiative called "Healthy Smiles for Wisconsin." The goal of the Healthy Smiles for Wisconsin Coalition is that no child in that state should go without adequate oral health care, preventive services, or education. The organization has developed a planning guide for communities wanting to set up a Seal a Smile Program. The guide is free of charge and provides a step-by-step plan for starting a sealant program.[20]

Oral Health Education

Health education is the process of teaching people about health. The scope of health education may include educational activities for children, parents, policymakers, or health care providers. Educational programs are developed and presented in many different formats and settings.

Oral health education is a learning experience directed at helping people prevent oral disease. Oral health education can be presented directly to the clients through individual or group activities, such as health fairs, or in school curricula (Fig. 5–10). The intent of oral health education is to assist people in making decisions about their oral health and to choose behaviors conducive to maintaining this health.

For heath education to be effective, the participant must be actively involved in the learning process. The cognitive model alone (attitude + knowledge = behavior change) has been ineffective in producing change. The educator must consider many factors that influence learners and their behavior. Both internal and external factors should be considered in developing an oral health educational program (Fig. 5–11). Patient attitudes and environment affect behaviors and the possibility of change. The outcome of the oral health education process will be successful only if all factors are considered.

In regard to the sociodemographic factor of age, most dental education programs have been implemented for children. Oral health education for

Figure 5-10. Dental hygiene students use puppets to present oral health education at a health fair.

children is a priority because of the high prevalence of dental caries in this group. If a society free of dental disease is the goal, educational programs must be targeted for the future of society—the children. The school system, therefore, continues to be the setting utilized to implement large-scale oral health education programs. The school-based oral health education program remains an important component of the goal of optimal oral health for all citizens. Oral health education should be an integral component of all school health education curricula.

Other opportunities for oral health education can be accessed through faith-based, community-based, and social service organizations, such as the WIC Program, Head Start, Lions' Clubs, and Rotary Clubs. These

Figure 5-11. Factors influencing the dental education process. (Data from Web sites for state oral health programs.)

Individual factors (internal)

Education level
Beliefs, values, perceptions
Age, income, race, and other sociodemographic factors

Environmental factors (external)

Intrapersonal interactions with family and peers
Community influences, including cultural norms and
  public policy
Technology to deliver the information

organizations present opportunities for oral health education on a diversity of topics such as:

- Prenatal and postnatal oral health education for parents, infants, and toddlers
- Oral health concerns of special care patients
- Oral health education for older adults
- Oral health effects of tobacco and oral cancer information

Oral health educational programs can be given through health-care facilities, such as hospitals and clinics, and long-term care facilities, such as nursing homes and alternative care centers. Specialty groups such as the Four-H Club, Future Farmers of America, sports clubs, and youth organizations welcome educational programs. See Chapter 7 for additional information on health promotion.

State Oral Health Programs

Figure 5–12 presents a synopsis of the most common oral health programs offered in various states. The most common programs are in the areas of fluoridation, sealants, early childhood caries, health education and

Figure 5–12. Synopsis of state oral-health programs.

Access to Dental Care Programs
Prevent Abuse and Neglect through Dental Awareness (PANDA) Program
Children Forensic Identification team
• Community Dental Sealant Programs
Community Oral Health Systems Development
• Community Water Fluoridation
• Dental Screening Programs
• Early Childhood Caries and Baby Bottle Tooth Decay Programs
Fee-For-Service Programs for Indigent Children
Fluoride Supplement Programs
Head Start Grantees Reviews
Mouth Guard and Injury Prevention Programs
• Needs Assessment and Oral Health Surveys
Old Age Pensioners Dental Program
Oral Health Assurance
• Oral Health Education and Promotion Programs
Oral Health for School Nurses Program
Private Well Water Testing Program
• School Fluoride Mouth Rinse Programs
• Tobacco Cessation and Spit Tobacco Programs
Treatment Clinics and Mobile Dental Units

• The most common programs

promotion, and tobacco cessation.[21] Examples of successful programs in the fluoride arena and in the placement of sealants have been provided.

In the area of early childhood caries, the Texas Department of Health has implemented an oral health education program called "Take Time for Teeth." In this program, outreach workers, educators, and health care providers are taught a standardized oral health message that emphasizes preventive oral health practices at an early age. The people trained are chosen because they interact with the population targeted, that of children and families. Topics include:

1. Dental checkups for pregnant women.
2. Recognition of "white spots" and how to prevent baby bottle tooth decay.
3. The benefits of taking a child to the dentist every 6 months beginning at age 1 year.
4. The importance of dental sealants in preventing tooth decay.

The long-term goal of this statewide program is to have a positive impact on oral health status and to facilitate a positive behavioral change relating to oral health and prevention.[22]

A national tobacco cessation program is the National Spit Tobacco Education Program (NSTEP), funded by the Robert Wood Foundation and administered by the Oral Health America and supported by Major League Baseball. The goal is to educate young people on the dangers of using spit tobacco. Tobacco is presented as a potentially dangerous drug that can cause oral cancer. NSTEP and its partnerships with public, private, and voluntary groups, including the dental and medical professions, are helping Americans to stop using tobacco. The program uses television, radio, print, and public service announcements featuring baseball celebrities to send its message into the community.[23] For additional information on oral health programs, refer to the Web sites at the end of the chapter.

As oral health professionals, dental hygienists are educated to incorporate prevention and oral health education into every patient encounter. The dental hygienist in the role of Educator/Health Promoter uses the knowledge of primary preventive measures (e.g., fluorides, sealants, and oral hygiene care) to inform people on how to improve their oral health. Keeping updated on available resources and health education programs for special populations in the community assists the dental hygienist in the roles of Resource Person and Consumer Advocate.

SECONDARY AND TERTIARY PREVENTION PROGRAMS

Treatment Component

For better understanding of the impact of public health on dental disease, one must remember that dental diseases are not reversible and are not self-curing. Although primary preventive procedures are very successful in reducing the prevalence and incidence of the major dental diseases, prevention has not been able to eliminate them. Approximately 60% of Americans visit a dental office yearly. [24] Cost is a major reason why people do not see a dentist. People often wait to visit a dentist only in emergencies. Financial barriers and geographic access become reasons why people do not receive primary prevention and are thus in need of secondary or tertiary treatment of dental disease. Therefore, in addition to a preventive component, a treatment component is an essential element of a public oral health program.

Delivery of dental care in public health dental clinics can include fixed dental clinics, which may be run by federal, state, county, city, or private not-for-profit organizations. The practice of clinical dentistry in the public health setting is also accomplished through mobile clinics (vans), or with the use of portable dental equipment (see Chapter 2). Secondary and tertiary levels of prevention include the treatment of dental disease for people of all ages and with diverse backgrounds.

Services for Older Adults

An expanding population in need of both primary prevention and secondary and tertiary care is the elderly in our communities. Between 1990 and 1994, the number of older adults increased 11-fold (from 3 million to 33 million). These people are now the fastest-growing segment of the population in the United States. The U.S. Census Bureau projects that the number of persons aged 65 and older will more than double, by the middle of the 21st century, to approximately 80 million. In 1994, one in eight Americans were over 65 years of age; by the year 2030, one in five are expected to be in this category.[25]

The elderly not only are living longer but also are keeping their natural teeth; they are therefore in need of dental services and a means to pay for the services. As the income of older people declines with retirement, insurance programs eliminate the dental component for persons over 70 years and Medicare does not cover dental services. In the role of Change Agent and Consumer Advocate, dental hygienists can actively participate in supporting legislation to include dental as a component of health care for the elderly.

An example of a program for elderly dental care at reduced cost is the "Apple Tree Geriatric Dental Program." Apple Tree provides both primary educational services along with secondary restorative treatment and tertiary services that include making and fitting partials and dentures. This program began in Minnesota in 1986, when a few dental professionals recognized the problems of access to care in the aging population. The program was initiated in an effort to bring oral health to older adults. The program works with state and local authorities to establish mobile sites and to seek funding sources for dental care. The program has expanded to include patients with special needs, children with disabilities, and indigent families. Apple Tree Programs are located in Minnesota and in North Carolina. More than 95 locations are available where numerous dental professionals provide oral health care to persons with special needs.[27]

With the growing elderly population, it is apparent that there is a need for more community oral health programs similar to Apple Tree and a need for dental professionals to study the social, demographic, health and economic characteristics of today's elderly citizens.

FINANCING PROGRAMS

The financing of public oral health has gone through transitions during the 1990s and will continue to change in the future. The change, it is hoped, will include expanding services to various population groups.

At present, funding for programs addresses the health issues of women and children and is accomplished through numerous federal initiatives. These public programs are concerned with the health and well-being of pregnant women and children; they not only cut across multiple agencies but also have multiple federal and state funding streams. The private sector and the business community work with state governors on initiatives that strive to improve health status and strengthen families. Public financing programs for oral health care are defined in Figure 5–13.[27]

Federal Initiatives

Federal initiatives that provide funding to states for programs addressing women and children's oral health issues include:

- Maternal and Child Health Services Block Grants (Title V)
- Special Supplemental Nutrition Program for Women, Infants and Children (WIC)
- State Children's Health Insurance Program (S-CHIP) through Title XXI
- Medicaid (Title XIX)
- Administration for Children and Families (ACF)

Block Grants

Maternal and Child Health Services Block Grants (Title V grants) provide funding to states for the provision of prenatal care for women, primary and preventive care for children, and health and supportive services for children with special health care needs.

Women, Infants, and Children's Program

The WIC program provides grants for supplement foods, health care referrals, and nutritional education for low-income pregnant, breast-feeding, and non–breast-feeding women in addition to infants and children found to be at nutritional risk.

Program	Explanation
• **Medicaid** (funded jointly by federal and state governments)	Comprehensive dental services for children under the Early and Periodic Screening, Diagnosis, and Treatment (EPSDT) program.
• **State Children's Health Insurance Plan** (funded jointly by federal and state governments)	Provides no direct legislative mandate for dental services but supports the inclusion of oral health care in each state's program.
• **Medicare** (funded by federal government)	Medical Insurance program for the elderly that does not cover dental care except when dental services are directly related to the treatment of the medical condition.
• **Head Start** (funded by federal government)	The dental component of Head Start includes mandated screening and referrals for necessary care. Some programs also provide fluoride treatments and pay for dental care for children who are not covered by Medicaid. All programs require that the children brush their teeth after eating meals provided by Head Start.

Figure 5–13. Public financing of oral health care.

State Children's Health Insurance Plan

CHIP provides funding through Title XXI grants to develop comprehensive health insurance coverage for children not covered by Medicaid or other third-party health insurance. CHIP provides for oral health services as well as traditional medical services.

Medicaid

Medicaid, or Title XIX, is a joint state-federal financed program that is administered by the states to provide medical assistance for the poor. In many states the Medicaid program has ventured into the Managed Care health arena in an effort to reduce health care expenditures while maximizing preventive health measures.

Administration for Children and Families

ACF, an agency of DHHS, is responsible for 60 programs that provide assistance to needy children and families, including the administration of the Medicaid program. Head Start, another program under ACF administration, serves approximately 800,000 preschool children annually. Head Start provides for medical as well as oral health screening and treatment of conditions identified for enrolled children. It also includes daily oral hygiene activities and weekly oral health curricula.

The provision of oral health services to individuals who fall outside the eligibility guidelines for entitlement programs, such as Medicaid, are often addressed through voucher or fee-for-service programs. These may be administered by state health departments, by state dental associations, or through private entities. Many of the fee-for-service programs provide for emergency oral health services for school-aged children. These programs use *nominators*, who are generally school nurses or social workers and are familiar with the economic status of the families seeking services. Although the initiation of the fee-for-service program is generally due to an emergent cause, providers are encouraged to try to meet all of the oral health needs of the patient within the guidelines of the program.

Donated Dental Services Program

The Donated Dental Services (DDS) Program also addresses the oral health needs of medically compromised, permanently disabled, or elderly people. This program is a joint effort of participating dentists, dental laboratories, and coordinating personnel. It provides one-time, comprehensive oral rehabilitation for qualifying individuals. Begun in Colorado, the DDS Program is branching out into other states as participating providers are identified.

Summary

The various community oral health programs introduced in this chapter offer practicing dental hygiene health care professionals an extension of their private practice experience. Becoming acquainted with the oral health care needs of the community at large—in conjunction with an understanding of the available program and funding resources from the local, state, and national levels—provides an opportunity for dental hygienists to have a positive impact on the overall health of their communities. In this manner, dental hygienists serve their profession, colleagues, and patients as Educators, Change Agents, and Consumer Advocates, providing leadership and increased understanding of the relationship between oral health and the health of the community as a whole. Additional resources are available through the Web sites listed at the end of the chapter.

APPLYING YOUR KNOWLEDGE

1. Research and prepare a report on fluoride concentration levels in existing water supply sources in your community.
2. Have a classroom debate on fluoridation. Appoint people to take pro and con positions, and research your position before the debate. Have a mock city council decide the outcome.
3. Develop a community oral health educational program. Write your goal and measurable objectives. Show all stages of development, including assessment, planning, implementing, and evaluating of the program.
4. Discuss how you, as a private practice dental hygienist, might help implement the core essential public health functions and oral health services in your community.
5. Research the possibility of forming an oral health coalition in your community. Whom would you invite to join the organization? Decide on the goals and objectives of the organization.

Dental Hygiene Competencies

Reading the material in this chapter and participating in the activities of Applying Your Knowledge will contribute to the student's ability to demonstrate the following competencies:

Community Involvement

CM.2   Provide screening, referral, and educational services that allow clients to access the resources of the health care system.

CM.3   Provide community oral health services in a variety of settings.

CM.5   Evaluate reimbursement mechanisms and their impact on the patient's or client's access to oral health care.

CM.6   Graduates will be able to evaluate the outcomes of community-based programs and to plan for future activities.

Health Promotion

HP.1   Promote the values of oral and general health and wellness to the public and organizations within and outside the profession.

HP.2   Evaluate factors that can be used to promote patient or client adherence to disease prevention and/or health maintenance strategies.

References

1. Institute of Medicine Committee for the Study of the Future of Public Health, Division of Health Care Services: A Vision of Public Health in America: An Attainable Ideal. In The Future of Public Health. Washington, DC, 1988, National Academy Press.
2. Oral Health in America: A Report of the Surgeon General, Rockville, Md: U.S. Department of Health and Human Services, National Institute of Dental and Craniofacial Research, National Institutes of Health, 2000.
3. Association of State and Territorial Dental Directors: Guidelines for State and Territorial Oral Health Programs, 1997.

4. Children's Alliance: Washington State Oral Health Coalition. Available from *http:/www.childrensalliance.org/teeth/Washington.htm* (accessed August 20, 2000).
5. Zarkowski P: Community Oral Health Planning and Practice: Comprehensive Review of Dental Hygiene, 4th ed. St. Louis, Mosby–Year Book, 1998.
6. Cormier PP, Levy JI: Community Oral Health. New York, Appleton-Century-Crofts, 1981.
7. Mann ML: Planning for community dental programs. In Gluck GM, Morganstein WM (eds): Jong's Community Dental Health, 4th ed. St. Louis, Mosby–Year Book, 1998.
8. Newbrun E: Effectiveness of water fluoridation. J Public Health Dent 49:279–89, 1989.
9. Centers for Disease Control and Prevention: Achievements in Public Health, 1900–1999: Fluoridation of drinking water to prevent dental caries. MMWR Morb Mortal Wkly Rep 48(41): 933–940, 1999. Available from *http://www.cdc.gov/epo/mmwr/preview/mmwrhtml/ mm4841a1. htm* (accessed August 24, 2000).
10. Community and other approaches to promote oral health and prevent diseases. In Oral Health in America: A Report of the Surgeon General. Rockville, Md, U.S. Department of Health and Human Services, National Institute of Dental and Craniofacial Research, National Institutes of Health, 2000.
11. Heller KW, Sohn W, Burt BA, Eckiund SA: Water consumption in the United States in 1994–96 and indications for water fluoridation policy. J Public Health Dent 59: 3–11, 1999.
12. Indiana State Department of Oral Health: Oral Health Programs. Available from *http://www.state.in.us/isdh/programs/oral/fluoride.html* (accessed August 30, 2000).
13. California Department of Health Services: Oral health programs. Available from *http://www.caphe.state.co.us/fc/oralhealth/oralhom.asp*) (accessed August 30, 2000).
14. Fluoridation Facts: Dietary Fluoride Supplement Schedule, 1994. Available from *http//:www.ada.org/consumer/fluoride/facts/tables.html*
15. Allukian M Jr, Horowitz AM: Effective community prevention programs for oral diseases. In Gluck GM, Morganstein WM (eds): Jong's Community Dental Health, 4th ed. St. Louis, Mosby–Year Book, 1998.
16. Helfenstein U, Steiner M: Fluoride varnishes (Duraphat): A meta-analysis. Community Dent Oral Epidemiol 22:1–5, 1994.
17. Milgram P, Reisine S: Oral health in the United States: The post-fluoride generation. Annu Rev Public Health 21:403–36, 2000.
18. Horowitz HS: Why I continue to support community water fluoridation. J Public Health Dent 60:67–71, 2000.
19. Healthy People 2010: National Health Promotion and Disease Prevention Objectives. Atlanta, Centers for Disease Control and Prevention, Health Resources and Services Administration, National Institutes of Health, 1999.
20. Healthy Smiles for Wisconsin: Available at *http://www.healthysmilesforwi.org/sealasmile.htm* (accessed August 26, 2000).
21. Centers for Disease Control and Prevention (CDC): Synopsis of State Oral Health Departments. Atlanta, CDC, Association of State and Territorial Dental Directors, 2000.
22. Texas Department of Health: Take Time for Teeth, Division of Oral Health. Available from *http://www.tdh.state.tx/dental/ttfthome.html*
23. Oral Health America: National Spit Tobacco Education Program (NSTEP). Available from *http://www.nstep.com* (accessed August 30, 2000).
24. Center for Disease Control and Prevention: National Center for Health Statistics. Fastats A to Z, updated January 19, 2000. Available from *http://www.cdc.gov/nchs/fastats/dental.-html* (accessed August 24, 2000).
25. Hobbs FB: The Elderly Population. U.S. Census Bureau. Available at *http://www.census.gov/population/www/pop-profile/elderpop.html* (accessed August 26, 2000).
26. Apple Tree Dental Program: Available from *http://www.appletreedental.com* (accessed August 30, 2000).
27. Bailit H, Edelstein B, Tinanoff N: Public financing of dental care: Impact and policy implications. J Dent Educ 63:882–886, 1996.

Web Sites for State Oral Health Programs

Arizona Department of Health Services
(*http://www.hs.state.az.us/cfhs/ooh/index.html*)

California Department of Health Services
(*http://dhs.cahwnet.gov/mcs/psd/omds/
omdsindex.htm*)

Colorado Department of Public Health
and Environment
(*http://www.caphe.state.co.us/fc/oralhealth/oral
/hom.asp*)

Georgia Division of Public Health and
Environment
(*http://www.ph.dhr.state.ga.us/programs/oral/
index.shtml*)

Hawaii Department of Health
(*http://mano.icsd.hawaii.gov/doh/resource/
Healthy_Hawaii/opd_h224.htm*)

Idaho Department of Health and Welfare
(*http://www2.state.id.us/dhw/hwgd_www/ecic/
Start_Ea.htm*)

Illinois Department of Public Health
(*http://www.idph.state.il.us/about/ohw.htm*)

Indiana State Department of Health
(*http://www.state.in.us/isdh/programs/oral/
fluoride.html*)

Iowa Department of Public Health
(*http://www.idph.state.ia.us/fch/dh.htm*)

Louisiana Department of Health and
Hospitals
(*http://www.tulane.edu/~oralhlth/oral.htm*)

Maine Department of Human Services
(*http://www.state.me.us/dhs/ddh/index.htm*)

Maryland Department of Health
(*http://mdpublichealth.org/oralhealth/*)

Massachusetts Department of Public
Health
(*http://www.state.ma.us/dph/ooral.htm*)

Missouri Department of Health
(*http://www.health.state.mo.us/Aboutthe
Department/DS7.htm#DentalHealth*)

Montana Department of Public Health
and Human Services
(*http://www.dphhs.state.mt.us/hpsd/pubheal/
healsafe/dental/*)

Nebraska Health and Human Services
System
(*http://www.hhs.state.ne.us/deh/dehindex.htm*)

New York State Department of Health
(*http://www.health.state.ny.us/nysdoh/aids/
manuals/children/ped_chlb.htm*)

North Carolina Department of Health and
Human Services
(*http://www.community/health.dhhs.state.nc.
us/dental.htm*)

North Dakota Department of Health
(*http://www.health.state.nd.us/ndhd/prevent/
mch/oralhlth.htm*)

Oregon Department of Human Resources
(*http://www.omap.hr.state.or.us/providerinfo/
orprovguides/*)

Pennsylvania Department of Health
(*http://www.health.state.pa.us/floride.htm*)

Tennessee Department of Health
(*http://www.state.tn.us/health/oralhealth/*)

Texas Department of Health
(*http://www.tdh.state.tx.us/dental/dental.htm*)

Virginia Department of Health
(*http://www.vdh.state.va.us/fhs/dental/
    dental.htm*)

Washington State Department of Health
(*http://www.doh.wa.gov/cfh/*)

West Virginia Department of Health and
    Human Resources
(*http://www.wvdhhr.org/bph/hp2000/oral.htm*)

Wisconsin Department of Health and
    Human Services
(*www.healthysmiles.forwi.org/*)

Research

6

Stacy Long, RDH, MS

OBJECTIVES

Upon completion of this chapter, the student will be able to:

- Differentiate between the hypothesis and the null hypothesis of a research study
- Explain the importance of the scientific method in research
- Define a population and a sample as related to research
- Discuss sampling techniques and their uses
- Discuss the difference between the independent and dependent variables
- Use the terms mean, median, and mode to express the results of data collection
- Define the terms continuous and discrete data and their respective scales of measurement
- Discuss the uses of various statistical techniques
- Use different types of displays to exhibit data
- Explain the difference between type I and type II errors
- Define probability and statistical significance
- Express the importance of evaluating dental literature
- Explain the criteria for reviewing scientific literature
- Review a scientific journal article relating to dentistry

Key Terms

Hypothesis	Convenience Sampling	Mode
Null Hypothesis	Experimental Group	Range
Calibrated	Control Group	Variance
Validity	Independent Variable	Standard Deviation
Reliability	Variable	Correlation
Interrater Reliability	Dependent Variable	Parametric
Intrarater Reliability	Data	Normal Distribution
Population	Continuous Data	*t*-Test
Parameter	Discrete Data	ANOVA
Target Population	Interval	Nonparametric
Sample	Ratio	Chi-Squared Test
Statistic	Nominal	Power Analysis
Pilot Study	Ordinal	*P* Value
Random Sampling	Descriptive Statistics	Type I Error
Stratified Sampling	Inferential Statistics	Type II Error
Purposive (Judgmental) Sampling	Mean	Refereed
	Median	Abstract

Opening Statement

Questions in Research

♦ *How does a public health team decide that fluoridation in a community's water supply will reduce the incidence of new carious lesions?*

♦ *Exactly how much fluoride is required to add to the water to achieve a therapeutic effect without a toxic reaction?*

♦ *How would officials determine that dental hygienists might improve the quality of life in older people if they were able to work independently in extended-care facilities?*

♦ *How do communities decide to spend money on a program providing dental care to individuals with human immunodeficiency virus (HIV) infection instead of to children with special disabilities?*

♦ *Where can dental hygienists readily find employment, and what salary can they expect to earn?*

QUESTIONS AND ANSWERS IN RESEARCH

Although dental hygienists may seek the answers to the questions in the Opening Statement, patients may have other concerns, for example:

- Does a particular mouth rinse really reduce plaque buildup?
- Which brand of toothpaste is best?
- Can nonsurgical periodontal therapy provide results comparable to a those of a surgical procedure?

Even though students may commonly learn the answers to these questions from instructors or colleagues, it is important to understand where to find reliable answers to these questions independently as well as to understand the process that provides these answers.

Research via the scientific method is the basis from which these answers are produced. Manuscripts published in reputable scientific journals disseminate the results of independent research. To determine whether the information contained therein is indeed reliable and valid, certain knowledge and skills must be a part of the repertoire of every competent dental hygienist practicing in the dental community. This chapter provides a basic outline of what research entails and a method of evaluating the results of that research.

THE SCIENTIFIC METHOD AND DEVELOPMENT OF A RESEARCH PROBLEM

Understanding the basics of research entails gaining an appreciation for the components of a good research study, that is, understanding how a research idea is formulated, how a study is designed and executed, and how the resulting data are critically evaluated so that one can infer appropriate conclusions. Research can be thought of as a search for truth as well as the knowledge gained from this search. A true definition of research is a systematic inquiry that uses orderly scientific methods to answer questions or solve problems.[1]

The discoveries provided by research may lead to new knowledge or to the revision of existing knowledge. Dental research involves a systematic search for knowledge about issues relevant to the profession. To increase the chance that research will be valid, reliable, and relevant, the *scientific method*—a series of logical steps starting with the formulation of a problem—is employed (Fig. 6–1).

Formulation of a Problem (Asking the Question)

The first step in beginning a research study is the formulation of an idea. The idea is usually formed from a question that has been raised by a

> • Formulation of a problem (asking the question)
> • Formulation of a hypothesis (a proposed answer to the question)
> • Collecting the data (finding existing information related to the question as well as gathering of your own information)
> • Analysis and interpretation of the results
> • Presentation of the results
> • Formulation of conclusion (relationship of results to hypothesis)

Figure 6–1. The scientific method.

researcher. The question may arise from a very simple observation or thought. For example, during the clinical phase of dental hygiene education, participants might debate about the following:

1. Which areas of the mouth are most difficult to probe accurately?
2. What are the effects of diet on periodontal disease?
3. How can adequate oral health care be maintained by physically and mentally challenged people?

From simple notions such as these, a research question or problem can be formulated.

Examples of a research problem formulated from the previous questions might be as follows:

1. Which quadrant in the human dentition is least accurately probed by the second-year dental hygiene student at University X when using the Periodontal Screening Record (PSR) method of probing?
2. What is the percentage of calories from carbohydrates in the diet of patients exhibiting class II periodontal disease?
3. What effect does modifying the brushing techniques of disabled patients in long-term care facilities have on the gingival bleeding index of these patients?

The research problem should be kept as simple and concise as possible. A successful study often depends on an uncomplicated research design, which results from simple questions.

Formulation of a Hypothesis (A Proposed Answer to the Question)

After a research question is formulated, the next step is the development of a **hypothesis**, a statement that reflects the research question. The hypothesis is stated in positive terms that represent the researcher's prediction or opinion. An example of a hypothesis for the question "Which quadrant in the human dentition is least accurately probed by the second-year dental hygiene student at X University when using the PSR method of probing?" would be as follows: Second-year dental hygiene students at University X using the PSR method are most inaccurate when probing the distal lingual surface of teeth in the upper right quadrant of the mouth.

The research statement is often expressed as a **null hypothesis**, which assumes that there is no statistically significant difference between the groups being studied. An example of a null hypothesis for the preceding question would be as follows: Second-year dental hygiene students at University X show no difference in the accuracy of probing any tooth in the mouth when using the PSR method.

Once the hypothesis has been formed, data can be collected to prove or disprove the statement.

Collecting Data (Finding Existing Information and Gathering Information Independently)

After a research idea and a hypothesis are initially identified, the relevant available literature is reviewed. By examining an area of general interest, the researcher may be inspired to create a research question to resolve unknown or unexplained portions of the area of interest. Alternatively, when a general topic has been selected, a literature review may help to bring the topic into sharper focus. Emulating the accepted research designs that have been previously validated by others, the researcher can then design a study to evaluate the idea. Analysis of the literature is described later in this chapter.

After review and analysis of the available literature, the researcher can plan how the study will be conducted and how the data will be collected. Many different techniques can be used to collect data (see Chapter 3). During data collection, it is important to use **calibrated** instruments that are both valid and reliable. When examiners are involved in data collection, it is imperative that they be calibrated (i.e., in agreement with a set standard of performance for the data collection). For example, if one examiner notes caries on the occlusal surface of a first molar, a second examiner should also be able to note caries on the occlusal surface of the same first molar.

Validity is concerned with gathering data that have been intended to be collected. For example, if two calibrated dentists are examining children for occlusal caries on first molars, both dentists must examine and record caries only on the occlusal surfaces and only on first molars. They are examining the correct surfaces and collecting data that were intended to be collected.

Reliability refers to the consistency and stability of the data. The data are reliable if the examiners are calibrated and can reproduce the results. Both examiners must find the same three occlusal caries on first molars in child No. 1. If they examine child No. 1 an hour later, they should still find the same three occlusal caries as detected previously.

Interrater reliability refers to two or more examiners being in agreement with their findings. **Intrarater reliability** refers to one examiner being consistent with the findings previously recorded by the same examiner.

In developing the plan for conducting the study, it is important to identify the characteristics of the group involved in the study. Group characteristics are defined by such terms as population, sample, experimental, and control. The term *data*, or information, collected from the study group is defined and used in different ways. These terms and their relationship to the collection of research data are explained next.

Population and Sampling

POPULATION

Population can be defined as the entire group or whole unit of individuals having similar characteristics from which the results of an investigation can be inferred.[5] In regard to numerical characteristics of the population, the term **parameter** is used.

Populations can be very large or very small, depending on the topic to be studied. For example, in the first research question (which quadrant in the human dentition is least accurately probed by second-year dental hygiene students at University X using the PSR method of probing?), one can infer that the total population consists of second-year dental hygiene students. It would be optimal to examine each of these students to arrive at the answer. The second-year dental hygiene students are also known as the **target population,** or the population from whom the information is being collected. Because of time constraints, lack of resources, or financial issues, however, it may be decided that a smaller group within this group can provide the researchers with a significant result.

SAMPLING

Taking a portion of the population is known as *sampling*. A **sample** is a portion or subset of the entire population that, if properly selected, can provide meaningful information about the entire population. When one is discussing numerical characteristics of samples, the term **statistic** is used.

Samples can be large or small and are chosen to most appropriately reflect the research being done. A large sample usually provides the most accurate representation of the population and increases the exactness and accuracy of the data collected. Occasionally, a small sample may be used, as in the case of data collection for a **pilot study**, or trial run, done in preparation for a major study.

The importance of using a sample becomes obvious in regard to our research question. Suppose there is an urgent need to refine teaching techniques for probing and there is not enough time to adequately assess each second-year dental hygiene student's probing at University X. The researcher may thus decide to use only a portion, or sample, of the first-year class.

If it is decided that a sample of the population is to be used, different techniques are used to choose the sample. There are several types of sampling.

Random Sampling. The method of sampling that provides the most *external validity*, or degree to which the results of the study can be generalized to settings other than the one included is called **random sampling.** This method provides a sample in which each member of a population has an equal chance of being included and is the procedure of choice because it prevents the possibility of selection bias by the researcher.

As an example, assume that all second-year dental hygiene students at University X have been given a number. There are 50 students in the second-year class, and it is determined that a sample of 10 students will participate in the research. Numbers 1 to 50 would be written on separate slips of paper and placed in a container. From the container a number is drawn. The number is noted as one of the 10 students to be used in this sample. That number is then placed back in the container, and another selection is made until the list of 10 numbers is complete. The importance of placing each number selected back into the container is to preserve a true random selection from 50 numbers. Numbers that are drawn more than once are put on the list only once and are again placed back in the container.

Stratified Sampling. What if probing discrepancies are unique to the university's dental hygiene program? A random sample may not accurately assess the problem for all second-year dental hygiene students; it may be necessary to include students from other universities as well in a method called **stratified sampling.** Subdivisions of a population with similar characteristics, such as second-year dental hygiene students attending different dental hygiene programs, are called *strata*. The random selection of subjects from two or more strata of the population is another way of defining stratified sampling.

Systematic Sampling. Another form of sampling, **systematic sampling,** involves the selection of subjects by including every *nth* person in a list. For example, if a researcher had a list of second-year dental hygiene students by number and chose every odd-numbered person, he or she would be sampling the population systematically. In this case, unless the list is in random order, not every person may have an equal or random chance of being selected; thus, systematic sampling may not be considered a true random sample.

Purposive (Judgmental) Sampling. If an instructor who most often works with students who are learning probing techniques chooses the sample, it is easy to imagine that a great deal of bias may be introduced into the study. **Purposive,** or **judgmental, sampling** provides a sample, through personal judgment, of subjects that would be most representative of the population.

Convenience Sampling. A convenience sample may also introduce bias. Selection of a sample through **convenience sampling** provides a group of individuals who are most readily available to be subjects in the study. For example, a researcher conducting the probing study might enroll only individuals from the researcher's university as subjects.

Experimental and Control Groups and Variables

EXPERIMENTAL AND CONTROL GROUPS

After the sample population is selected, subjects may be divided randomly into experimental and control groups, which are used to answer a research question posed when an experimental treatment or manipulation is imposed on the research setting. The **experimental group** is the sample group in a study who receives the experimental treatment or intervention. The **control group** is the group in a study who does not receive the experimental treatment or intervention. The control group provides the baseline against which the effects of the intervention on the experimental group can be measured.

For example, let us assume that the study on probing accuracy did find an area of the mouth where inaccuracy predominated. At this point, one might chose to conduct another research study, introducing a new method of probing instruction that would focus on the area of the mouth where most inaccuracies occur. This new method of teaching would be administered to the experimental group, whereas the control group would continue to receive the traditional method of instruction.

VARIABLES

The experimental treatment or intervention that is imposed on the experimental group can also be called the **independent variable**. A **variable** is a characteristic or concept that varies, or is different, within the population under study. The independent variable is controlled or manipulated by the researcher and is believed to cause or influence the **dependent variable**. The dependent variable is thought to depend on or to be caused by the independent variable. It is the outcome variable of interest.

In the case of the research question, which involves teaching a new probing technique to the experimental group, the dependent variable would be probing accuracy. The independent variable would be the probing technique that is being taught. Other variables not related to the purpose of the study are *uncontrolled* variables and may influence the relationship between the independent and dependent variable. To increase *internal validity,* it is important to control for extraneous variables. Internal validity refers to the fact that it is the experimental treatment or independent variable that is responsible for the observed effects and that these effects are not due to extraneous variables. A good research study controls for extraneous variables through research design or through statistical procedures.[6] By understanding the previous terms and definitions, one can implement a method of data collection, or the gathering of information, to address a research problem.

Data

Pieces of information, such as numbers collected from measurements and counts obtained during the course of a research study, are known as **data**. Although the concept of data itself may seem fairly straightforward, there are actually several different types of data as well as ways to measure data:

1. **Discrete data** have only one of a limited set of values and are counted only in whole numbers. Discrete variables may include things like hair color, gender, political preference, and number totals, such as how many times a person brushes his or her teeth or the number of decayed, missing, or filled teeth. These data are considered to be *qualitative* in nature.
2. **Continuous data** are measurements made from a particular value within a defined range. Variables along a continuum, such as temperature, scores on a test, and time, are continuous data. These data are considered to be *quantitative* in nature.

Different scales of measurement are used for discrete and continuous data. Discrete data can use nominal or ordinal scales of measurement. Continuous data use interval and ratio scales of measurements.

Nominal scales of measurement consist of named categories with no order. For example, females may be placed in category A and males in category B.

Ordinal scales of measurement consist of categories of variables in which the categories are in order but there is no equal or defined distance between them. For example, the American Academy of Periodontology (AAP) classification of periodontal disease is a subjective judgment of disease with categories of type I, type II, type III, and type IV. It is known that type II is worse than type I and that type III is worse than type II, but by how much is not defined.

Interval scales of measurement have equal distance between variables, but there is no true zero point (i.e., temperature on a Fahrenheit thermometer).

Ratio scales of measurement have equal intervals between the variables but there is a meaningful zero point (i.e., height and weight).

As listed next, each scale of measurement takes on the characteristics of the previous one, making ratio the most powerful measurement:

Nominal: named categories only
Ordinal: same as nominal plus categories are in order
Interval: same as ordinal plus equal intervals between categories
Ratio: same as interval plus meaningful or true zero point

After the data have been collected from a chosen population and variables have been defined as well as measured, it is time to proceed to the next step of the scientific method, presenting and interpreting the data and presenting the results.

Data Analysis and Presentation of Results

Statistics

Statistics is a science that provides a way of processing numbers or analyzing the data that have been collected. Statistics may be used to describe, analyze, and interpret the numbers collected in the data. The purpose of statistical analysis is to make an inference or an assumption about a population. Two types of relevant statistics are as follows:

1. **Descriptive statistics** are used to describe and summarize data. Their objective is to communicate results, without generalizing beyond the sample, to any population. Some ways in which results are communicated are through (a) *measures of central tendency* (mean, median, mode) and (b) *measures of dispersion*.
2. **Inferential statistics** (see later) are used to apply information from the sample to a larger population.

Measures of Central Tendency

Measures of central tendency are used to describe the sample based on the data gathered. They include components such as the mean, median, and mode.

The **mean** is the average of the group. It is a sum of all the values divided by the number (n) of items and is statistically noted as $\bar{x}$. The mean is calculated in the following manner:

$$\text{mean} = \frac{\Sigma \bar{x}}{n}$$

The positive aspect of the mean is that it includes the value of each score; the negative aspect is that it can be affected by any extreme scores and may not give a true average. For example, a test is administered; 10 people in the class score an 85 and 2 people score a 30. The class average becomes approximately 76, which is not a true representation of the class scores.

The **median** represents the exact middle score or value in an ordered distribution of scores; it is the point above and below which 50% of the scores lie. When the total number of scores is even, the sum of the two middle scores, divided by 2, provides the median.

Unlike the mean, extreme scores do not affect the median. In the previous example, the median score would be 85. However, it is not difficult to imagine what would happen if scores were not evenly distributed and the median were used as an example of the middle score. The information provided in this case may not demonstrate a true midpoint for the class.

The **mode** is the score or value that occurs most frequently in a distribution of scores. Once again, the mode for the preceding example would be 85. The distribution of scores may be unimodal, bimodal, or multimodal, or there may even be no mode.

Figure 6–2 presents the mean, median, and mode of a group of test scores. Figure 6–3 illustrates a symmetric distribution in which the mean, median, and mode are the same; it also shows skewed curves, where the mean and median are located to the left and right of the mode.

Measures of Dispersion

In addition to the measures of central tendency (mean, median, and mode), measures of dispersion (also known as measures of variation) may also be used to describe data. Measures of central tendency provide a first

Figure 6–2. Graph of student test scores.

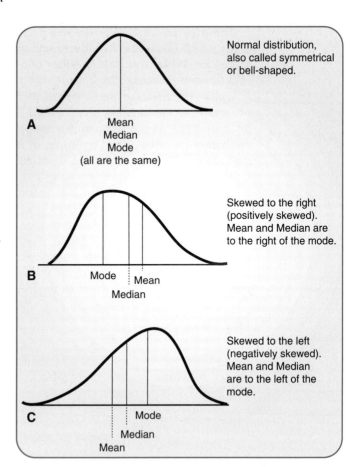

Figure 6–3. *A–C*, Graphing measures of central tendency.

step in the measure of distributions. Occasionally, however, a measurement is also desired to determine how far scores differ from the mean.

The most obvious way of measuring the dispersion of data is the **range**, which measures the difference between the highest and lowest values in a distribution of scores. If the median is defined as the point where 50% of the scores are lower and 50% of the scores are higher, the location of the 0 and 100th percentile would define the range. More commonly, the value of the range is used to define the 5th and 95th percentiles. These are the points that 5% of the subjects may be below or 95% of the people may be below. If a person has taken a test and is in the 95th percentile, 95% of the people have scored lower than that person has.

Another measure of dispersion, called **variance,** is a method of ascertaining the way individual variables are located around the mean. Variance is most often used to measure interval and ratio variables.

A first step in the calculation of variance is to determine the average deviation, which can be derived through calculating the difference between each point of data and the mean, adding the answers together, and

dividing by the total amount of data points. The main problem with calculating the average difference is that there are as many negative data
points as positive; this situation ultimately results in an answer of zero.

A way around this is to square each data point so that all terms are
positive. Therefore, the difference between each data point and the mean
squared, summed, and divided by the total amount of data points results
in the average squared deviation, also known as variance.

Variance is simply a step in determining the standard deviation (SD)
and is equal to the square of the SD. The formula for the SD is as follows:

$$SD = \sqrt{\frac{\text{sum of (data point} - \text{mean)}^2}{\text{No. of values}}}$$

It makes sense, then, that the farther away the data points are from the
mean, the greater the variance and SD. Figure 6–4 presents the calculations to find the range, variance, and SD of student test scores.

Figure 6–5 demonstrates the calculations from data collected in a community research project involving unwed teenaged mothers and their
knowledge of baby bottle tooth decay. There are 12 mothers in this study
group. The mother's scores from the pretest range from a low score of
25% to a high score of 70%.

Correlation

After we determine the previous information about our data, we may
want to next determine whether any **correlation** exists between the variables. Correlation is a statistical method for determining whether a variation in one variable may be related to a variation in another variable. For
example, height and weight often show a correlation, since taller people
usually have a higher weight than shorter people. Age and periodontal
disease may have a correlation, since older people may have higher incidence of periodontal disease than younger people.

The technique used to determine correlation depends on the type of
variable being explored. Different techniques are used for discrete or continuous variables. The measurement scale may also influence the technique. For example, nominal, ordinal, interval, and ratio scales of
measurement are all calculated slightly differently.

The results of the calculation for correlation show either a negative or
positive relationship. When the relationship is *positive*, it is predicted that
as the value of one variable increases, the other also increases. Perfect
positive correlation is shown by +1.0. An example would be the finding
that, in the research with unwed mothers, the more time the examiner
spends with them on patient education, the greater the increase in the
mothers' knowledge. Table 6–1 presents a correlation of increased education with increased knowledge. Figure 6–6 demonstrates a graphic display of the same positive correlation of the two variables.

Student test scores

Number of students	Score
6	60
3	30
3	100
4	45
4	95
5	90
5	50

Range is the difference between highest and lowest score: 100 − 30 = 70

Variance is the average deviation or spread of scores around the mean. The variance is calculated as (individual score − mean)^2/# of scores.

$(60 − 67)^2 = 49$
$(30 − 67)^2 = 1369$
$(100 − 67)^2 = 1089$
$(45 − 67)^2 = 484$
$(95 − 67)^2 = 784$
$(90 − 67)^2 = 529$
$(50 − 67)^2 = 289$

49 x 6 (# of scores of 60) = 294
1369 x 3 (# of scores of 30) = 4107
1089 x 3 (# of scores of 100) = 3267
484 x 4 (# of scores of 45) = 1936
784 x 4 (# of scores of 95) = 3136
529 x 5 (# of scores of 90) = 2645
289 x 5 (# of scores of 50) = 1445

All above summed = 16,830

16830 ÷ 30 (total number of scores) = 561

561 is the variance

Standard deviation is the positive square root of the variance: $\sqrt{561}$

The square root of 561 = 23.7 (standard deviation)

Figure 6–4. Range, variance, standard deviation of student test scores.

In contrast, a *negative* correlation shows an inverse relationship between variables. Perfect negative correlation is shown by −1.0. Figure 6–7 shows that a diet including six servings of fruits and vegetables each day *decreases* the incidence of certain cancers.

In review, a perfect positive correlation is noted as +1.0 and a perfect negative correlation showing an inverse relationship is noted as −1.0 Although a perfect positive or perfect negative correlation may occur, it may be possible to find no relationship at all; this instance is noted as 0.0. Some literature

Subject (mother)	Score (%)
1	45
2	45
3	45
4	30
5	35
6	25
7	40
8	50
9	60
10	65
11	70
12	70

Median = 45%
Mode = 45 %
Mean = 48%

Range = 70 − 25
= 45

$$\text{Variance} = \frac{\text{sum of (individual scores − mean)}^2}{\text{\# of scores}}$$

= 210

Standard deviation = $\sqrt{210}$

= 14

Figure 6–5. Calculations of test scores on baby bottle tooth decay.

states that generally a correlation coefficient above .70 is considered satisfactory.[1] In each study, the nature of the variables and the numbers involved in the comparison must also be considered along with the correlation coefficient in determining what is a significant relationship. The closer the relationship is to +1.0 or −1.0, the more perfect, or stronger, the correlation.

Table 6–1
Correlation of Test Scores and Hours of Education

Group No.	Group Type and Pretest Scores	Hours of Education	Average Post-Test Score Increase (Points) %
1	Four mothers with an average pretest score of 50	2	60
2	Four mothers with an average pretest score of 50	4	70
3	Four mothers with an average pretest score of 50	6	80
4	Four mothers with an average pretest score of 50	8	90

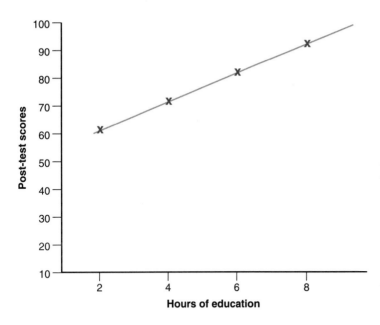

Figure 6-6. Post-test scores and hours of education (positive correlation).

Presentation of the Data

In addition to the data displayed in the previous graphs, other types of data display include the following:

A *bar graph* is most often used to display nominal or ordinal data that are discrete in nature. Using data that may be gathered from the study on

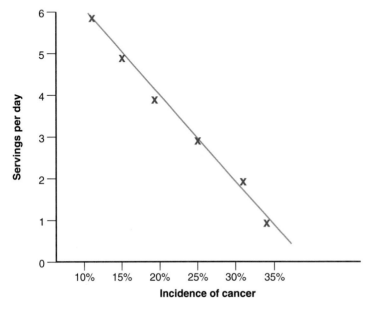

Figure 6-7. Number of fruit and vegetable servings per day related to percent incidence of cancer (negative correlation).

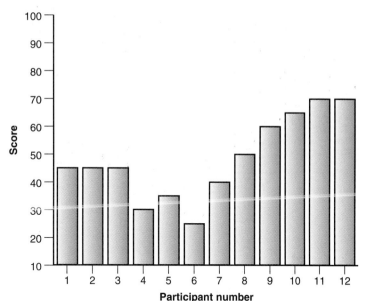

Figure 6–8. Pretest scores of 12 participants as shown in a bar graph.

teenaged mothers and baby bottle tooth decay, one can create a bar graph to present the data pictorially (Fig. 6–8).

A *frequency polygon* is used to represent data that are continuous in nature. An example from the study with teenaged mothers is depicted in Figure 6–9. The figure contains dots connected to straight lines to present the frequency distribution of the data. In this case, the frequency polygon

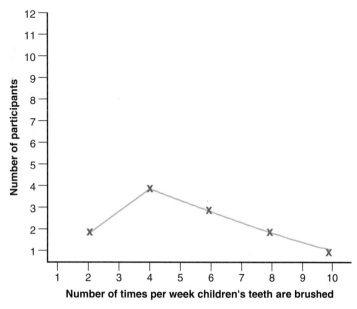

Figure 6–9. Number of times per week participants brush their children's teeth as shown in a frequency polygon.

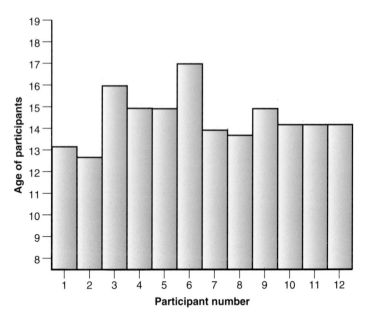

Figure 6–10. Age of 12 participants in the research study as
shown in a histogram.

demonstrates how many times per week the mothers brush their children's teeth.

A *histogram*, although a type of bar graph, is used most often to represent interval or ratio scaled variables that are continuous in nature (Fig.
6–10). The bars in a histogram are of equal width and touch each other to
indicate that the data are being presented on a continuum.

Inferential Statistics

In addition to including descriptive techniques to describe data, inferential statistics may also be used. Whereas descriptive statistics are used to
determine information only about the sample being studied, inferential
statistics seek to determine a generalization between the sample studied
and the actual population. The larger the sample size, therefore, the
greater the number of generalizations that can be made regarding the
population. Depending on the type of data collected, the use of inferential
statistics may include either parametric or nonparametric statistical techniques. Inferential statistics are based on the assumption that sampling is
conducted randomly, although that is not always the case.

Parametric Inferential Statistics

Parametric statistics are used when the data include interval or ratio
scales of measurement. Parametric techniques work best when the sample
is large and randomized and the population from which the sample is

taken is normally distributed. In a normal distribution, 50% of the values lie on the left half of the distribution and 50% lie on the right half. A **normal distribution** assumes that approximately 68% of the population fall within one SD of the mean, approximately 95% fall within two SDs of the mean, and 99% lie within three SDs from the mean.[9] The plotting of these data on a graph results in a bell-shaped curve (Fig. 6–11).

t-TEST

Parametric statistics are calculated by means of several different methods or tests. One of the most common is the *t*-test, or Student's *t*-test, so named for the man responsible for development of this technique. The *t*-test is used to analyze the difference between two means. It provides the researcher with the difference between treatment and control groups or groups receiving treatment A versus treatment B.

When the test is used on a single group who yields pretreatment and post-treatment scores, it is known as a *t*-test for *dependent samples*. This test analyzes data when only one independent variable is tested. For example, a researcher may want to examine the difference in blood glucose levels of diabetic subjects before and after treatment with a new diet. Assuming that all of the subjects were the same age and had the same degree of disease present, the *t*-test for dependent samples can be used to determine pretreatment and post-treatment scores.

The *independent* *t*-test determines differences in the mean between two independent groups, such as an experimental and control group or males versus females. This test is used when only one or two independent variables are tested. Most often, data involving interval or ratio scales of measurement are statistically analyzed with an independent *t*-test. For example, a study might investigate the effect of a new toothbrushing method on gingivitis. The subjects would be randomized into two groups: (1) a *control* group receiving no instruction and asked to use their normal

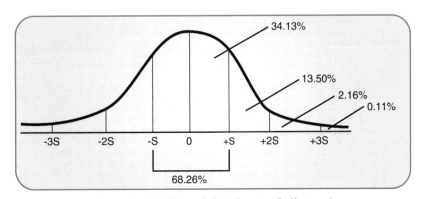

Figure 6–11. Normal distribution (bell curve).

brushing method and (2) an *experimental* group asked to practice a new method of toothbrushing. The instrument may be a gingival bleeding index that is conducted before the start of the study and again 8 weeks later. The hypothesis is that the new method of toothbrushing will decrease the gingival bleeding index of patients with gingivitis.

ANALYSIS OF VARIANCE (ANOVA)

Another commonly used test for parametrics is **analysis of variance,** or **ANOVA**. This test allows comparison among more than two sample means and compares interactions among the variability in the multiple sample groups with the variability within the groups.

A simple example is the comparison of the many brands of desensitizing toothpaste. Five brands of toothpaste that claim relief of tooth pain due to sensitivity have been located. A group of subjects is assembled, and each subject is given a different toothpaste disguised in a plain white tube. Each subject is asked to use this tube and is given other tubes to use until all of the various toothpastes are used. Subjects are asked to rank pain relief from tooth sensitivity on a numerical scale of 1 to 10 for each toothpaste used. The scale may look like the one in Table 6–2.

ANOVA allows the dental hygienist to compare each toothpaste used and the pain relief experienced by the patients. It also allows a comparison of the different responses from each patient for each individual toothpaste brand. ANOVA may yield information about which of the brands is actually more effective and how each brand compares with another. In essence, ANOVA compares variability *within* groups with variability *between* groups.

The *t*-test, or Student's *t*-test, and ANOVA are just two of many tests that may be used in statistical analysis of data. These tests are perhaps the most common parametric inferential statistical techniques.

No matter which technique is chosen, the sample should be randomly and independently selected from normal populations. Although these

Table 6–2 Data Used in Analysis of Variance (ANOVA) Testing					
Patient No.	TP-1	TP-2	TP-3	TP-4	TP-5
1	6.0	5.0	4.0	5.0	2.0
2	5.0	5.0	3.0	4.0	3.0
3	7.0	5.0	4.0	5.0	3.0
4	5.0	4.0	4.0	3.0	4.0
5	6.0	5.0	5.0	4.0	4.0

TP, toothpaste brands 1 to 5.
Key: 1.0–10 = pain relief (10 is maximum relief).

tests provide more detailed information of the interaction of variables, the research should include means and SDs in the report for accurate assessment of the tests' magnitude.

Nonparametric Inferential Statistics

Besides parametric tests, **nonparametric** inferential statistical techniques may be selected. Nonparametric techniques are most useful for data to be measured on the nominal or ordinal scale. Remember, nominal or ordinal data are "qualitative," and although numbers may be included, these numbers are derived more subjectively than numbers associated with quantitative data. Nonparametric tests involve fewer assumptions about the population. The sample size may be small, and variables are discrete.

The most commonly used nonparametric test is the **chi-squared test**. This test may be used to analyze questionnaire data and to determine whether a relationship exists between two variables. The chi-squared test is used to examine the differences between observed and expected frequencies.

Determining Statistical Significance

Statistical tests provide researchers with an idea of what the data they have collected say about the sample and perhaps what the data imply about the population from which the sample was drawn. An important factor in research is determining the statistical significance of the data. Statistical significance is a way of indicating that the results found in an analysis of data are unlikely to have been caused by chance; more likely, the results have been caused by the independent variable. Using too small or too large a sample may influence the statistical significance. Typically, the use of too small a sample (less than 30) provides too little information to make generalizations about the populations and to create any significance of results.

POWER ANALYSIS

Determining how many subjects are needed to provide significance is called a **power analysis**, which is calculated according to a specific statistical formula based on what the researcher hopes to observe in the majority of subjects. The *power* of a study, or its ability to detect relationships among variables, is directly related to sample size, the definition of the independent variable, and the precision with which the study is planned and conducted.[10] When too large a sample is used, the effects may be statistically significant but clinically of no consequence.

The true importance of determining statistical significance is that the greater the significance, the more statistical inference can be made regarding the population from whom the sample was taken. That is, statistical significance reinforces our ability to generalize the conclusions we make about our study population to a larger population, perhaps even to the "general population."

A major issue in regard to statistical inferences is that every measurement taken from the sample being researched has some degree of error. Researchers may describe the possibility of error or lack or error in various ways.

CONFIDENCE INTERVALS

The term *confidence interval* refers to how researchers describe the probability of the statistical results being correct. A confidence interval indicates a range of values within which the parameters of the population have a probability of lying. Researchers usually use a 95% to 99% confidence interval. A 95% confidence interval indicates a probability that the researcher is wrong 5 times in 100. By using a 99% confidence interval, the researcher may be wrong 1% of the time; however, increasing the confidence interval also decreases the specificity of the data. Therefore, when the confidence interval is 95%, there is a 5% chance that the observed results or differences between study and control groups are due purely to chance and not a true difference caused by the independent variable.

P VALUES

Researchers also use **P values** to describe statistical significance. The P value states how likely it is that the study could have come to a false scientific conclusion. P values are calculated according to the sample size, the difference between the means of the control and experimental group, and the SD of the distribution. The smaller the P value, the more significant the findings of the study are considered.

A normally acceptable P value is $P < .05$. Results with a P value at less than .05 are generally considered statistically significant and provide the basis for rejection of the null hypothesis $P < .05$ means that the results were due to chance only 5 times in 100. P values of approximately .01, .001, and lower increase the significance of the study.

Formulation of a Conclusion and Relationship of Results to the Hypothesis

Based on the statistical results of the data analysis, the researcher determines whether the study shows significance. Whether it shows much, little, or no significance, a conclusion can be formulated. From the results

		Null hypothesis is:	
		Accepted	Not accepted
Null hypothesis is actually	True	No error	Type I error α (alpha)
	Not True	Type II error β (beta)	No error

Figure 6–12. Null hypothesis.

discovered, the researcher decides to either accept or reject the null hypothesis of the study. Occasionally, when formulating a conclusion, a researcher may make an error. Errors within research are of two types:

Type I alpha (α) errors occur when, according to statistical results, the researcher rejects the null hypothesis when it is true. The researcher's conclusion states that a relationship exists when it does not. Most statistical analyses use an α level of .05, which means that there is a 1 in 20 chance that a conclusion will state that a difference exists when there is no difference.

Type II beta (β) errors occur when the null hypothesis is accepted but is actually false. The conclusion states that no relationship exists when one actually does (Fig. 6–12).

▧ ANALYSIS OF THE LITERATURE

A thorough review of the literature is often completed in order to begin development of an adequate plan for collecting the data. Being informed and up to date not only are professional responsibilities but also serve a purpose in each of the six contemporary roles of the dental hygienist: Clinician, Educator, Manager, Change Agent, Consumer Advocate, and Researcher.[2] The assimilation of information requires more than listening to colleagues and attending occasional Continuing Education programs. An excellent source of information is dental and other scientific literature.

A literature analysis, besides helping the dental hygienist to develop a data collection plan, provides valuable information about theories, methods, and products that are available. Reviewing the literature is an important step in remaining current within the field of dentistry and provides information used to intelligently answer many questions posed by patients. Scientific literature contains information that can help one to maintain competency and helps to set the exceptional practitioner apart from others in the field of dentistry.

Not all dental hygienists receive regular subscriptions to scientific magazines or have access to Internet services. Although these are the most common ways to obtain information about literature, a trip to a local library with a scientific collection can provide essential information. Becoming skillful at obtaining scientific information is not as easy as might be expected. However, it is a skill worth cultivating because it provides a valuable tool for researchers as well as for practicing dental hygienists.

The topic described next presents an overview of what is available in the form of written resources, how to choose the best sources of this information, and how to critically review this literature. Although a critical analysis of the scientific literature is ideal, it is best to remain open-minded when inquiring about new products, services, and techniques.[3]

Finally, keeping focused on the research or specific information to be reviewed should help to provide simple yet intelligent answers to the question at hand.

Selection of Literature

To begin a literature review, the dental hygienist or researcher must select appropriate journals. The scientific writing to be reviewed should be comprehensible to the average dental hygienist who is knowledgeable about the topic area. The selection of literature that is pertinent to the field of dental hygiene will allow the researcher to obtain a complete understanding of the research topic while focusing the research on issues important to dental hygiene. Because of the technicality and intricate scientific detail of its topics, the *Journal of Biochemical Research* might not be an ideal place to start looking for information on periodontal host factors, whereas the *Journal of Periodontology* and *Journal of Dental Hygiene* might be preferable choices. Although both journals publish in-depth scientific literature, the material is tailored to the dental field and thus is relevant and understandable to the average oral health researcher.

Of equal importance is the selection of a reputable journal. Several aspects lend credibility to a reputable source, including an editorial review board that evaluates each contributed article for accuracy, relevancy of content, and issues involving style and method of scientific writing. This is also known as a **"refereed,"** or a *"peer-reviewed"* journal. Individuals who are considered experts on the article's content review the articles submitted with a peer review board. A refereed journal ensures that an article is written in appropriate scientific style and that the data published therein reflect current knowledge. A reputable journal is commonly affiliated with a professional group or society, a specialty group, or a reputable scientific publisher. A reputable scientific journal is not a journal that is a popular magazine or published by a commercial firm.

Examples of poor choices for scientific literature include any of the typical newsstand health and recreation journals as well as glamour and beauty magazines. Professionals should appreciate the fact that although there are many attractively presented dental publications, many are simply glorified advertising brochures and do not represent an acceptable source of scientific material. When selecting a journal article, the reader should be careful to note that the author has the appropriate qualifications. (An attorney writing an article about orthodontics, for example, might not be the most credible source of information.) Authors should also possess experience or a current relationship with the field about which they are writing. If the written work is a research study, there should be evidence of facilities in which to conduct the research as well as financial support for the project.

Readers usually find a tremendous amount of available information. Although older information may be considered classic and therefore occasionally useful in conducting a review, most often readers want to research the most current information. One classic study was the Vipeholm study, conducted in Sweden in the 1950s.[4] The study investigated the incidence of decay in relation to sugar intake and is often mentioned in scientific writing. Although the information from this research has proved valuable, this study was conducted in a disadvantaged population and by today's standards would not have received approval because of ethical considerations. One of the most often cited concerns about the Vipeholm study was whether the subjects enlisted possessed the mental capacity to give their consent for the research.

Information is usually considered current if it has been published within the last 3 to 5 years. References cited in journal articles should be carefully screened to validate their relevancy and age. Sometimes only a limited amount of information is available on a given topic, and this is reflected in the article. An example is the lack of true research involving herbal or alternative dental therapies.

Evaluation of the Selected Literature

After a journal and the information relevant to the reader's goals are selected, the reader can pursue a comprehensive evaluation of this literature. Various types of journal articles undergo different types of review. For example, a *review article* may examine an assortment of studies that have already been conducted and provides an overview of the research that has already been done. A review article can help one formulate an idea or a new research question and can help direct the reader to other sources of information through references cited within the article. Validation of a good review article should follow all of the practices stated earlier, including author expertise, accurate and recent references, and review from a refereed journal.

The Primary Research Manuscript

Perhaps the most useful type of journal article and truly the archetypal "research paper" is the primary research manuscript (Fig. 6–13). A primary research study describes the original research, including its methods, materials,

A. Abstract
- Contains 200 words or less.
- Clearly states purpose of study in the first few sentences.
- Includes brief description of the following: population, type of research, overview of statistics, results and conclusions.

B. Introduction
- Review of the supporting literature.
- Statement of hypothesis (null hypothesis).
- Reason for study.

C. Methods and materials
- Appropriate selection of instrument.
- Appropriate method of conducting research (i.e., prospective, retrospective, randomized, etc.).
- Descriptive enough that reader can replicate the study.

D. Results
- Appropriate statistical tests.
- Appropriate display of data.
- Clear and understandable presentation of the data.
- Correct interpretation of data.

E. Discussion
- Conclusions are based on fact.
- Results are tied into previous research discussed in introduction.
- Inferences and opinions are stated as such.
- Future plans are included for further research.

Figure 6–13. What to look for in a research study manuscript.

results, and conclusions. When one is considering a primary research article, the practice of checking author expertise, accurate and recent references, and peer review from a refereed journal still applies; additionally, other steps are to be followed. The first step is often an assessment of the paper's abstract.

Abstract

A relevant **abstract** is usually confined to approximately 200 words and concisely defines the study's purpose, methods, materials, and results. The abstract, a brief description of the research, appears at the beginning of the manuscript and is designed to provide the reader with an overview of the study. Although it may present an idea of what the study involved, the abstract may not always paint an accurate picture of the study and the results. The only way to truly assess a scientific article is to read the content within and critically examine each piece for information.

A primary research article begins with a review of the current literature and an introduction to the study. Within this section, an accurate and complete description of the research problem is given and the purpose of the study is clearly stated. The research question can be stated as a hypothesis and may include objectives to be accomplished.

Materials and Methods

The next section of the primary research manuscript, materials and methods, describes the population or sample and the techniques used to gather information about the population studied. One of the primary reasons for disseminating results in peer-reviewed journals (in addition to sharing the results) is so that colleagues might duplicate the experiment to validate the results or might modify it in some respects to further refine the conclusions implied in the study. Toward that end, the materials and methods text should be complete enough so that other readers might reasonably expect to recapitulate the experiment and verify the results.

The reviewer will want to determine whether or not the researcher has selected an appropriate group to test and whether it is one that is relevant to the reviewer's needs. This necessity for appropriateness applies whether the "group" in question is a population of laboratory animals, human subjects, or tissue culture cells. For example, if reviewers are looking for information regarding nonsurgical periodontal therapy, they should ensure that the study has used a similar population or sample relative to their needs.

The number of subjects in the group is also important. Has the study included enough subjects so that readers can generalize the findings to their group of interest? If the subject is a 35-year-old woman and the research involves men older than 50 years of age, the results may not necessarily be relevant to the reader's cause; if the subject is a 35-year-old woman but only one or two subjects are involved, the information might also be irrelevant.

Ensuring that no author *bias* has been introduced is very important. Bias may be defined as any influence that produces a distortion in the results of a study.[1] Here are some considerations:

- Is the subject a patient of the researcher, who also happens to be the one who developed the new technique?
- Are all variables in the study controlled for (e.g., diet, standard of living, gender, age, dental history)?
- Is there a control group and an experimental group?
- Is one group receiving the standard treatment and the experimental group receiving the new therapy?

An example of a research study may be the evaluation of the efficacy of sealants in caries prevention. The study design may consist of a group of test subjects (the experimental group) who are to receive sealants and are then to be monitored for a number of years to determine the caries rate. Since reference data are essential, a control group (the group without sealants) is compared with the group with sealants.

Readers must also consider the following issues when evaluating research design:

- If an instrument (e.g., a questionnaire) is to be part of the study, have validity and reliability been previously established?
- Are the conditions under which the treatment is accomplished similar and completely described?
- Are both groups monitored for an adequate period of time to assess long-term results of the therapy?

Results

After the methods and materials are described, the results section, including a statistical analysis, follows. The results text should detail how the hypothesis of the study has been tested. Statistical tests should be appropriate for the study and should be described. Tables and graphs may be included to provide a visual representation of the results, but they should be clear and understandable to the reader. The author should justify the statistical method used.

Discussion

Finally, a discussion of the conclusions and the inferences drawn from the results of the research is presented. The conclusions are also used to define outcomes of the research.

The conclusion should clearly state the rejection or acceptance of the null hypothesis. It may discuss facts derived from the research but may also include investigator speculation on what the results mean. The conclusion usually discusses the research study's strengths and weaknesses and may mention further research necessary to obtain the desired results.

Complications observed during the research should also be presented. The results of the study are related to the literature cited. Most important, the conclusions are a direct reflection of the findings. Although speculation may be appropriate, it should be stated as such. It is never appropriate to make statements that are not based on fact or that are not derived from study results.

Summary

This chapter has provided an overview of the basics of research, including the steps in the scientific method, the steps in analyzing the literature, and the components of a primary research manuscript.

Although all research should be conducted according to the scientific method to provide results with a measure of validity and reliability, scientific research remains an inexact science. However, when studies are properly designed and accurately analyzed using the appropriate statistical design, the information obtained not only will be new but also may serve as a springboard for further studies. The inventive and inquisitive practitioner will seek to discover information that both enhances the practice of dental hygiene and all its contemporary roles and keeps the profession moving in a forward direction.

APPLYING YOUR KNOWLEDGE

1. Formulate a research problem based on a question you have that is related to the field of dentistry.
2. Develop a hypothesis and a null hypothesis for the research problem.
3. Considering your research problem, define the following:
   a. Population
   b. Sample
   c. Experimental group
   d. Control group
   e. Independent variable
   f. Dependent variable
4. Determine whether the data collected from your study will be continuous or discrete. Will nominal, ordinal, interval, or ratio scales of measurement be used?
5. Complete a literature review for the research problem formulated in No. 2, and write an abstract for one of the journal articles examined during your literature review.
6. Using data that you have reviewed or collected, determine the mean, median, and mode.
7. Give five examples of positive and negative correlations. Compare variables related to dental hygiene or to data from articles you have read.
8. Using one of the research studies from your literature review, describe the statistical analysis. Were the statistical techniques used appropriate? Were the data displayed in an appropriate manner?
9. Design and complete a research study or community project following the steps listed in Figure 6–1 (the scientific method). Complete your study by creating a poster presentation using appropriate displays of data and the description of your study.

Dental Hygiene Competencies

Reading the material in this chapter and participating in the activities of Applying Your Knowledge will contribute to the student's ability to demonstrate the following competencies:

Core Competencies
C.4 Assume responsibility for dental hygiene actions and care based on scientific theories and research as well as the accepted standard of care.

Community Involvement

CM.6 Evaluate the outcomes of community-based programs, and plan for future activities.

Patient/Client Care

PC.1 Systematically collect, analyze, and record data on the general, oral, and psychosocial health status of a variety of patients or clients using methods consistent with medicolegal principles.

PC.3 Collaborate with the patient, client, or other health professionals to formulate a comprehensive dental hygiene care plan that is patient-centered and based on scientific evidence.

References

1. Polit D, Hungler B: Nursing Research Principles and Methods, 5th ed. Philadelphia, JB Lippincott, 1995.
2. Darby M, Walsh M: Dental Hygiene Theory and Practice. Philadelphia, WB Saunders, 1995.
3. Hittleman E: Analysis of the dental literature: More accessibility through informatics. In Gluck GM, Morganstein WM (eds): Jong's Community Dental Health, 4th ed. St. Louis, Mosby–Year Book, 1998.
4. Gustafsson BE, Quensel CE, Swenander LL, et al: The Vipeholm Dental Caries Study: The effect of different levels of carbohydrate on caries activity in 436 individuals observed for five years. Acta Odont Scand 11:232–364, 1954.
5. Monsen E: Research: Successful Approaches. Chicago, American Dietetic Association, 1992.
6. Norman G, Streiner D: PDQ Statistics. Philadelphia, BC Decker, 1986, p 15–18.
7. Zarkowski P: Community Oral Health Planning and Practice: Comprehensive Review of Dental Hygiene, 4th ed. St. Louis, Mosby–Year Book, 1998.
8. American Academy of Periodontology. Proceedings of the World Workshop in Clinical Periodontics, Princeton, NJ, July 23–27, 1989.
9. Rose L: Introduction to biostatistics. In Gluck GM, Morganstein WM (eds): Jong's Community Dental Health, 4th ed. St. Louis, Mosby–Year Book, 1998.
10. Potter P, Perry A: Research in nursing care. In Contemporary Nursing: Dimensions and Dynamics. St. Louis. Mosby–Year Book, 1993.

Bibliography

Armstrong RL: Hypothesis formulation. In Krampitz SD, Pavlovich N (eds): Readings for Nursing Research. St. Louis, CV Mosby, 1981.

Campbell JP, Draft RL, Hulin CL: What to Study: Generating and Developing Research Questions. Beverly Hills, Calif, Sage Publications, 1982.

Huff D: How to Lie with Statistics. New York, WW Norton, 1954.

Kleinbaum DG, Kupper LL, Morganstern H: Epidemiological Research. Belmont, Calif, Lifetime Learning Publications, 1982.

Kraemer LG: Research and theory development in dental hygiene. In Darby ML, Walsh MM (eds): Dental Hygiene Theory and Practice. Philadelphia, WB Saunders, 1995, p 1109.

Norman GR, Streiner DL: PDQ Statistics. Philadelphia, BC Decker, 1986.

Polit DF, Hungler BP: Nursing Research: Principles and Methods, 5th ed. Philadelphia, JB Lippincott, 1995.

Health Promotion and Health Communication

Beverly Isman, RDH, MPH

OBJECTIVES

Upon completion of this chapter, the student will be able to:

◆ Discuss various health promotion theories and their application to promotion of oral health

◆ Discuss the distinctions between "generic," "targeted," "personalized," and "tailored" health messages

◆ Identify strategies for delivering health information to consumer groups by using innovative visual materials and activities and methods for evaluating the effectiveness of the strategies

◆ Outline the basic components, advantages, and limitations of table clinics, poster presentations, oral papers, and round table discussions as methods of presenting scientific information to health professionals

◆ List examples of service-learning programs that can increase a dental hygienist's understanding of community dental health issues and approaches

◆ Identify professional organizations that offer opportunities for personal growth and development in the field of community health and dental public health

Key Terms

Health Promotion

Theories

Stages of Change Theory

Health Belief Model

Social Learning Theory

Community Organization
Theory

Diffusion of Innovations
Theory

Organizational Change:
Stage Theory

"Framing" Health Messages

"Tailoring" Messages

Focus Groups

Learning Styles

Quantitative Evaluation

Qualitative Evaluation

Table Clinic

Poster Presentation

Oral Paper

Round Table Discussion

Service-Learning Programs

Opening Statement

Challenges to Promoting Oral Health

◆ *Despite years of research on prevention of dental diseases, we know very little about how best to promote oral health.*

◆ *We need much more evidence that changes in attitudes and beliefs about oral health lead to improved oral health outcomes.*

◆ *Improved knowledge levels rarely translate into healthful behaviors.*

◆ *Most behavioral change that occurs after oral health education or promotion is short term and is not sustained without periodic reinforcement.*

◆ *Despite the lack of evidence of the effectiveness of oral health education and health promotion efforts to improve health, we ethically must disseminate scientific knowledge to the public.[1]*

◆ *Today dental hygienists have unique and unlimited opportunities to become involved in community health activities and to contribute to the development of a better understanding of effective oral health promotion efforts.*

▨ HEALTH PROMOTION THEORIES

The World Health Organization defines *health* as:

> the extent to which an individual or group is able, on the one hand, to realize aspirations and satisfy needs; and, on the other hand, to change or cope with the environment. Health is, therefore, seen as a resource for everyday life, not the object of living; it is a positive concept emphasizing social and personal resources, as well as physical capabilities.[2]

This view conceptualizes health as a personal resource and a lifestyle that should be promoted and introduces the role of behavior, not just knowledge, into the health equation. This chapter, therefore, focuses on the concepts of oral health promotion, behavior change, and the dental hygienist's role in communicating health messages to other health professionals and to the public.

Health promotion is a broad concept that refers to the process of enabling people and communities to increase their control over the determinants of health (see Chapter 3) and, therefore, to improve their own health. Health promotion goes beyond prevention of disease and reduction of health risks. Aspects of health promotion include:

1. Advocacy.
2. Efforts to change organizations, policies, and environments.
3. Political considerations.
4. Ethical responsibilities.

Oral health promotion efforts can increase demand for care, use of dental services, and preventive self-care measures. The anticipated outcome of these efforts is a reduced incidence and severity of oral diseases with improved oral health. Yet, as we see in the challenges in the Opening Statement, applied research relating to oral health promotion is still in its infancy and not well integrated or coordinated with research and theories developed by other health disciplines.

In the effort to promote health and prevent disease, **theories** help us to analyze and interpret health problems and then to plan and evaluate interventions. What is a theory?

A theory is a set of interrelated concepts, definitions, and propositions that present a systematic view of events or situations by specifying relations among variables, in order to explain and predict the events or situations.[3]

A theory is an abstract notion that comes to life only when it is applied to specific topics and problems. Sometimes theories are called *conceptual frameworks* or *models*.

How can you apply theories to dental hygiene practice and public health practice? Every day, dental hygienists face challenging situations that cause oral problems, such as patients who feed their babies cariogenic liquids in baby bottles, athletes who sustain oral injuries because they refuse to wear a mouth guard, and adults who say they are too busy to keep their recall appointment. Theories can help us to analyze these situations and to apply solutions that have been effective in similar circumstances.

Traditionally, dental hygienists have viewed oral health problems primarily as the "patient's" problem and have proceeded to "educate" the patient about how to improve oral health. This approach is doomed to failure because it does not assess or validate the patient's point of view and does not consider the environmental circumstances that have influenced the person's attitudes, knowledge, or health practices. It is important to analyze oral health problems from more than one perspective and to understand how each perspective affects the others. Behavior that leads to improved oral health can be affected at three levels:

- ◆ Intrapersonal (within the individual)
- ◆ Interpersonal (between people)
- ◆ Community (including institutional or organizational change as well as public policy)

The following section describes selected health promotion theories that relate to these three levels and that have the most relevance to oral health issues. Each explanation is accompanied by a table that contains key concepts, definitions, and applications of each concept to a problem. For easier reading, I have included texts that cover overviews of most of the theories in the References instead of citing the original references for the theories.[3, 4]

Intrapersonal Level

Stages of Change Theory (Transtheoretical Model)

Initially developed by Prochaska and DiClemente, the Stages of Change Theory views change as a process or cycle that occurs over time rather than as a single event. This theory allows the dental hygienist to assess a person's readiness to change a behavior toward a more healthful lifestyle, for instance, daily brushing to prevent gingivitis. The theory assumes that at any point in time everyone is at a different stage of readiness to make lifestyle changes and that people cycle through the various stages over time, depending on the behavior to be changed. The major stages of this model with definitions and applications are outlined in Table 7–1.

The cycle starts by increasing one's awareness of a problem (e.g., a person has gingivitis) to initiating behavior change (brushing effectively and using antimicrobial rinses), and progresses to maintaining motivation to continue preventive actions (returning in 3 months to check progress). To be effective in changing behavior, health messages and programs should be matched to an individual's current stage of readiness to change.

Health Belief Model

Originated by Rosenstock and others in the 1970s to explain people's use of preventive health services, the Health Belief Model allows us to assess perceptions of how susceptible one is to a health problem and if one

	Table 7–1	
	Stages of Change Theory	
	(Transtheoretical Model)	
Concept	**Definition**	**Application**
Pre-contemplation	Being unaware of problem; not having thought about change	Increase awareness of need for change; personalize information on risks and benefits
Contemplation	Thinking about change in the near future	Motivate and encourage to make specific plans
Decision/determination	Making a plan to change	Assist in developing concrete action plans or setting gradual goals
Action	Implementing specific action or plans	Assist with feedback, problem solving, social support, and reinforcement
Maintenance	Continuing desirable actions or repeating periodic recommended steps	Assist in coping, using reminders, finding alternatives, avoiding slips or relapses

Modified from Glanz K, Rimer BK: Theory at a Glance: A Guide for Health Promotion Practice. Bethesda, Md, National Institutes of Health, 1997.

believes that recommended preventive behaviors will result in less susceptibility. For example, does your father think that he is at risk for development of oral cancer because he smokes a pipe? Does he believe that limiting use of the pipe would reduce his oral cancer risk? The model also looks at perceived severity of a disease threat, benefits of taking a health action, and barriers to completing the action. Does your father believe that the effects of quitting pipe smoking are worse than the effects of oral cancer?

One application of the Health Belief Model is to develop messages that are likely to persuade people to make decisions to improve their oral health. The components of the model and some applications are shown in Table 7–2. The primary hypothesis is that increased perception of severity and susceptibility to a disease results in an increased probability of taking action. Perceived ability to take action and cues to action are important factors. Does your father believe he can quit smoking his pipe, and what reminders can you provide to support him?

Table 7–2 Health Belief Model		
Concept	**Definition**	**Application**
Perceived susceptibility	One's opinion of chances of getting a condition	Define population at risk and risk levels; personalize risk based on a person's features or behavior; heighten perceived susceptibility if too low
Perceived severity	One's opinion of how serious a condition and its sequelae are	Specify consequences of the risk and the condition
Perceived benefits	One's opinion of the efficacy of the advised action to reduce risk or seriousness of impact	Define action to take: how, where, when; clarify the positive effects to be expected
Perceived barriers	One's opinion of the tangible and psychological costs of the advised action	Identify and reduce barriers through reassurance, incentives, and assistance
Cues to action	Strategies to activate readiness	Provide how-to information; promote awareness, send reminders
Self-efficacy	Confidence in one's ability to take action	Provide training and guidance in performing action

Modified from Glanz K, Rimer BK: Theory at a Glance: A Guide for Health Promotion Practice. Bethesda, Md, National Institutes of Health, 1997.

Interpersonal Level

Social Learning Theory

The Social Learning Theory posits that people learn primarily in four ways:

1. Direct experience.
2. Vicarious experience, such as through the mass media.
3. Judgments voiced by others, such as testimony or promotions by experts.
4. Inferred knowledge.

The basic premise of this theory, developed by Bandera and sometimes known as the Social Cognitive Theory, is that people learn through their own experiences, by observing the actions of others, and by the results of these actions. Behavioral change is accomplished through the interaction of personal factors, environmental influences, and individual behaviors. Self-efficacy and self-confidence are important concepts. Table 7–3 lists the relevant definitions and applications of the major concepts.

An example of applying the Social Learning Theory to oral health is helping a single mother to feel confident about performing toothbrushing

Table 7–3 Social Learning Theory (Social Cognitive Theory)		
Concept	**Definition**	**Application**
Reciprocal determinism	Behavioral changes result from interaction between the person and the environment; change is bidirectional	Involve the individual and relevant others; work to change the environment, if warranted
Behavioral capability	Knowledge and skills to influence behavior	Provide information and training about action
Expectations	Beliefs about likely results of action	Incorporate information about likely results of action in advance
Self-Efficacy	Confidence in ability to take action and to persist in action	Point out strengths; use persuasion and encouragement; approach behavioral change in small steps
Observational learning	Beliefs based on observing others like oneself and/or visible physical results	Point out others' experience and physical changes; identify role models to emulate
Reinforcement	Responses to a person's behavior that increase or decrease the chances of recurrence	Provide incentives, rewards, praise; encourage self-reward; decrease possibility of negative responses that deter positive changes

Modified from Glanz K, Rimer BK: Theory at a Glance: A Guide for Health Promotion Practice. Bethesda, Md, National Institutes of Health, 1997.

for her young child by using techniques such as demonstration, watching a video, providing ongoing encouragement, and giving periodic feedback. When the mother gains some confidence in her skills, she then assists the child care workers and other parents at the day care center in learning these skills so that they can support each other and so that oral hygiene care becomes a daily activity for all of the children.

Community Level

Community Organization Theory

Community Organization Theory is the process of involving and activating members of a community or subgroup to identify a common problem or goal, to mobilize resources, to implement strategies, and to evaluate their efforts. People usually refer to this process as *empowerment*. This is a grassroots approach to health promotion, rather than a project that is initiated and conducted by health professionals. Table 7–4 outlines the key components.

To apply an example, consider the role of a church pastor and a congregation in oral health promotion. Church members notice that many of the elders have stopped coming to church suppers because they have lost their teeth and are embarrassed to eat in public. The pastor calls the dental school for help, and the congregation raises money to help defray the cost of examinations and dentures for the elders. Dental and dental hygiene student teams work together to assess each elder's needs and to fabricate and fit the dentures. They also discuss oral health, denture care, and the challenges of eating with dentures. Gradually, the elders begin to become comfortable eating and speaking with the dentures, and they resume their attendance at church suppers. The following year, the church leaders continue to work with the student teams to promote oral health to people of all ages within their parish.

Diffusion of Innovations Theory

Developed by Rogers, the Diffusion of Innovations Theory helps us assess how new ideas, products, or services spread within a society or to other groups, that is, how innovations are adopted. During the assessment, attention is directed to the characteristics of the innovation, the communication channels, and the social systems. Table 7–5 displays the components.

Use of dental sealants is a good oral health example. Researchers found that despite numerous clinical trials showing their effectiveness in caries prevention, adoption of sealants by practitioners proceeded slowly. Adoption occurred much sooner in public health clinics, where there was a critical need for effective caries-preventive measures and strong advocacy for the procedure, than in private dental offices, where patients had low caries rates, insurance companies did not reimburse for the service, and

	Table 7–4 Community Organization Theory	
Concept	**Definition**	**Application**
Empowerment	Process of gaining mastery and power over oneself or one's community to produce change	Give individuals and communities tools and responsibility for making decisions that affect them
Community competence	Community's ability to engage in effective problem solving	Work with community to identify problems, create consensus, and reach goals
Participation and relevance	Learners should be active participant and work starting "where the people are"	Help community set goals within the context of preexisting goals, and encourage active participation
Issue selection	Identifying winnable, simple, and specific concerns as focus of action	Assist community members in examining how they can communicate the concerns and whether success is likely
Critical consciousness	Developing understanding of root causes of problems	Guide consideration of health concerns in broad perspective of social problems

Modified from Glanz K, Rimer BK: Theory at a Glance: A Guide for Health Promotion Practice. Bethesda, Md, National Institutes of Health, 1997.

practitioners were wedded to the use of amalgams for managing rather than preventing dental caries. Over time, caries rates in occlusal surfaces declined dramatically in children who received regular care at the clinics, whereas caries rates remained stable in the children visiting private dental practices. Major educational efforts, policy changes regarding reimbursement, and advocacy efforts were used to eventually change attitudes and patterns of practice in the private sector, thus resulting in reduced rates of dental caries in all children in the community.

Organizational Change: Stage Theory

Organizations pass through a series of four stages as they initiate change (Table 7–6). In addition, organizational structures and processes influence workers' behavior and motivation for change.

Table 7–5 Diffusion of Innovations Theory		
Concept	**Definition**	**Application**
Relative advantage	The degree to which an innovation is seen as better than the idea, practice, program, or product it replaces	Point out unique benefits: monetary value, convenience, time saving, prestige, etc.
Compatibility	How consistent the innovation is with values, habits, experience, and needs of potential adopters	Tailor innovation to the intended audience's values, norms, or situation
Complexity	How difficult the innovation is to understand or use	Create a program, idea, or product to be easy to use and to understand
Trialability	Extent to which one can experiment with the innovation before a commitment to adopt is required	Provide opportunities to try on a limited basis (e.g., free samples, introductory sessions, money-back guarantee)
Observability	Extent to which the innovation provides tangible or visible results	Ensure visibility of results: feedback or publicity

Modified from Glanz K, Rimer BK: Theory at a Glance: A Guide for Health Promotion Practice. Bethesda, Md, National Institutes of Health, 1997.

To apply the Organizational Change: Stage Theory, we can consider a situation in which health educators asked the cafeteria staff in the hospital to offer healthier foods. A number of stages were involved in instituting the change (e.g., pricing different food items, looking at sample menus, announcing the new food items). Eventually, a larger percentage of employees began to select the new food options, thus eating healthier lunches. Soon they asked for a larger selection of these foods. The health educator and the cafeteria staff then worked together to distribute health-promoting recipes so that employees also were encouraged to make healthy food choices at home. This process not only resulted in institutional change but also created healthier lifestyles in the employees' families.

ACQUIRING NEW KNOWLEDGE

To use these theories effectively, dental hygienists need to acquire new information for assessing and changing people's health behaviors. In

Table 7–6 Organizational Change: Stage Theory		
Concept	**Definition**	**Application**
Definition of problem	Problems recognized and analyzed; solutions sought and evaluated	Involve management and other personnel in awareness-raising activities
Initiation of action	Policy or directive formulated; resources for beginning change allocated	Provide process consultation to inform decision makers and implementers of what adoption involves
Implementation of change	Innovation is implemented; reactions and role changes occur	Provide training, technical assistance, and aid in problem solving
Institutionalization of change	Policy or program becomes entrenched in the organization; new goals and values internalized	Identify high-level champion, work to overcome obstacles to institutionalization, and create structures for integration

Modified from Glanz K, Rimer BK: Theory at a Glance: A Guide for Health Promotion Practice. Bethesda, Md, National Institutes of Health, 1997.

addition, they need to keep abreast of innovative programs occurring in other professions and ways in which other health care systems address health problems. This information guides the approach selected to assess and change people's behaviors (see "Guiding Principles" next).

Guiding Principles

Knowledge Needed to Assess and Change People's Behaviors[5]

♦ Factors that are considered a risk for development of oral diseases and those factors that can be modified through preventive efforts at the primary, secondary, and tertiary levels

♦ How to assess a person's risk for development of oral diseases and other health problems

♦ The level of scientific evidence for and the extent of certainty of the effectiveness of various preventive measures

♦ Which categories of interventions yield the desired impact (e.g., personal behaviors, programs, societal and environmental modifications, policies)

Guiding Principles continued on following page

Guiding Principles   *Continued*

- ◆ Effective oral and written communication skills
- ◆ Ways in which innovations are diffused and ways of bringing about organizational change
- ◆ Ways to motivate people to access services and return for continuing care
- ◆ The structure of various health care systems and community-based organizations
- ◆ How to deliver effective services and education
- ◆ How to evaluate efforts (e.g., effectiveness, costs, access, quality, outcomes)

Some of the information may be learned during the dental hygiene educational process, whereas some may be acquired through experience and professional development. Resources for professional development are discussed later in the chapter. Let us now examine how to design health messages, specifically, how to frame and tailor them.

FRAMING HEALTH MESSAGES

Within the last decade, the field of health communications research and media advocacy has increased exponentially.[6] New forms of technology are changing our options for framing, delivering, and evaluating health messages for the public. The concept of **"framing" health messages** relates to the cues (e.g., sounds, symbols, words, pictures) that signal how and what to think about an issue. In the process of framing messages, an attempt is made to connect to people's values, beliefs, knowledge levels, and emotions. **"Tailoring" messages** relates to the specific cues used to make messages meaningful for a specific individual.

A fundamental error in many oral health education efforts is the assumption that increased knowledge will result in changes in behavior. Traditionally, oral health messages have been packaged as "generic" messages that cover a number of concepts and try to appeal to the greatest number of people. A typical brochure would cover brushing and flossing as well as use of fluorides, sealants, antimicrobials, and other preventive measures. It might also describe various diagnostic procedures, such as radiographs, periodontal probing, and microbial tests. This type of brochure is based on the assumption that dental hygienists should provide as much information as possible and that people will sort through the information to select the pieces that apply. Numerous research studies have shown that this assumption is not necessarily valid; the approach is not effective for changing behaviors, particularly in busy people or low-level readers.

Using a more focused approach, health professionals began to use "targeted" materials intended to reach a specific subgroup or population, usually based on demographic characteristics (e.g., older adults, African Americans). The assumption that underlies this approach is that a large number of people still can be reached and that homogeneity exists in the group to justify the messages and formats used. Subgroups, however, often represent very heterogeneous groups, thus reducing the effectiveness.

Another approach is to "personalize" messages. Many of these attempts, however, have used personal characteristics on a superficial level (e.g., a person's name), assuming that using a person's name will draw attention to the generic information that is presented. Mail promotions use this technique extensively because lists of consumers and health professionals can easily be purchased. Although this approach initially may have a motivating effect, the appeal soon is lost. A more effective way to personalize information, for instance in a brochure, is to highlight only the information and key messages that apply to the person who receives it.

The most effective way to reach individuals to increase their knowledge or to change behavior is to "tailor" messages.[7] These messages or strategies are intended to reach a specific person on the basis of characteristics unique to that person that were discovered through an assessment process. This is the basis of many computerized risk assessment/risk reduction programs in health care (e.g., heart disease, diabetes.) The technique can be applied to the formation of an individualized oral health plan based on risk assessment and primary prevention measures.[8] The assumption is that tailored messages provide a more meaningful and motivating strategy built on a person's specific input. Unfortunately, professionals sometimes try to tailor messages without going through the essential assessment process, only to find that their messages are ineffective.

EXPANDING COMMUNICATION FORMATS

Health promotion efforts often are viewed with skepticism by dental researchers, who equate them with random distribution of brochures and with no evaluation of behavioral change. As explained earlier in this chapter, health promotion theories go "beyond the brochure" and involve careful needs assessment and evaluation.

Consumer-Oriented Presentations

Before health information is provided to an individual or to a group, an assessment process is crucial. Depending on the audience and topic, a needs assessment can be accomplished through a literature review, informal observations or conversations, surveys, in-depth interviews, or focus group interviews. This process reveals important cultural beliefs, health practices, and knowledge levels that result in misconceptions, barriers to care, or stumbling blocks to behavioral change.

The use of **focus groups** is one effective method of assessment. Group interviews are conducted with 5 to 10 members of the intended target audience and last about 30 to 60 minutes. A moderator uses structured questions to guide the discussion. When developing or testing health messages or materials, the moderator can use one or more versions of the materials to ask questions such as:

- What is one message you remember from the video?
- Were there any messages that were confusing?
- Did you relate to the people in the video? How were they like you? Different from you?
- Was the video too short, just right, or too long?
- Should the video be accompanied by a handout that you can take home to help you remember the information?
- Would this video motivate you to ask about dental sealants for your child's teeth?

Focus groups are particularly useful for determining whether messages are at the appropriate language and literacy levels and whether they are culturally acceptable to the people in the group. Information about the appearance and appeal of materials is particularly important.[9]

A variety of resources are available for dental hygienists to use when designing and evaluating health messages. Examples of formats for presenting information are included in Figure 7–1. References in this chapter provide citations describing the benefits and limitations of these various formats.[10-12] Some of the formats can be combined to allow for differences in **learning styles** of the audience. Assessing learning styles of individuals is much easier than planning messages to reach a diverse group of people. As a guide, people usually remember:

- 10% of what they read
- 20% of what they hear
- 30% of what they see
- 70% of what they see and hear
- 90% of what they see, hear, and do

Hands-on, interactive multimedia formats are usually more effective for retaining knowledge than simply reading or listening to a message. This is true whether one is presenting information to the general public or to other health professionals.

On the basis of the findings from the needs assessment and the methods selected for health promotion activities, an evaluation plan can be designed before any interventions are started. Evaluation plans should be linked directly to the project objectives and should include measures to

> **VISUAL DISPLAYS**
> - Posters, flip charts, story boards, bulletin boards, fotonovelas, models
>
> **WRITTEN PROMOTIONS**
> - Newsletters, newspaper articles, model legislation, fact sheets, booklets, storybooks
>
> **AUDIOVISUAL MATERIALS**
> - Videos, public service announcements, Web sites, audiotapes, slide shows, multimedia presentations
>
> **INTERACTIVE FORMATS**
> - Songs, role playing, storytelling, puzzles or quizzes or games, theater or puppet shows, demonstrations, computerized oral camera, interactive computer programs, science experiments or science fairs, debates, simulations

Figure 7–1. Formats for presenting oral health information to the public.

determine short-term and long-term effectiveness. Evaluation measures help to determine effectiveness (see "Guiding Principles" next).

Guiding Principles

Questions to Determine the Effectiveness of Project Objectives[13]

- ◆ Has the intervention achieved the desired results? If not, why not?

- ◆ Should this intervention be continued in its current form?

- ◆ What messages or activities produce the best results?

- ◆ How can the intervention be improved?

- ◆ Can it be replicated successfully in other settings?

- ◆ Are the resources (e.g., people, money, materials) that were used reasonable and cost-effective?

Evaluation can occur during and after the intervention. Measures can be **quantitative** (e.g., *how many* people increased their knowledge of the causes of early childhood caries) or **qualitative** (e.g., *why* did people participate in the activity and *how* do they intend to change their parenting behaviors?) Evaluation plans do not always have to be complicated and do not always have to use sophisticated statistical analysis. The key is to try to evaluate your efforts. Examples of simple evaluation strategies are listed:

1. Ask five questions to assess parents' knowledge and attitudes about sealants before and after a school-based sealant program.
2. Provide healthy snack recipes to a day care center; follow up after 2 months to determine which snacks have been made for the children and which snacks the children seem to like the best.
3. Survey school soccer coaches before and after initiating an oral injury or mouth guard campaign to determine use of mouth guards during practices and games, changes in policies on athletic equipment, and barriers that have been (or have not been) overcome in the attempt to implement the campaign.
4. Survey members of a community to identify how many heard the radio public service announcement about oral cancer prevention, where and how many times they heard it, and whether they followed any of its recommendations.
5. Use a consumer satisfaction questionnaire in a clinic to determine whether the patients are receiving all of the health information they want and need in effective formats that answer their questions or concerns in a culturally appropriate manner.

Presentations to Health Professionals

The purpose of professional presentations is to deliver thought-provoking information to a group of health professionals in a short period of time in a clear, concise, and visually appealing format. Presentations generally focus on new research, programs, theories and ideas, clinical techniques, products or materials, career opportunities, educational techniques, policies or legislation, health care systems, or methods for disease prevention or detection. The information covers a specific topic with key messages highlighted and sources well documented.

Specific guidelines for presentations may vary by the sponsoring organization. When selecting a topic and format for a presentation, consider the following five questions (see "Guiding Principles" next).

Guiding Principles

Five Questions for Selecting a Topic and Format

◆ Who will be the audience? How large a group do I want to address?

◆ What is their level of knowledge or interest in my topic?

◆ What questions might they ask? Will I be able to learn new information related to my topic from some members of the audience?

◆ How much time will I need to cover my key points?

◆ What audiovisual materials will most enhance my key points?

Most presentations follow a sequence, such as:

- Introduction and Background
- Methods and Materials
- Findings/Results or Key Points
- Discussion and Significance
- Summary and Conclusions

To apply these principles to the area of community health, I next show a comparison of four common types of presentations at dental or public health meetings.

Presentation for a Table Clinic[14]

Note: The table clinic format is not used routinely outside the dental and dental hygiene professions.

Time: 5 to 7 minutes, occasionally 7 to 10 minutes

Format: Oral presentation by one or two people using audiovisuals that are placed on a table; same presentation is repeated a number of times for different groups

Size of Audience: Usually five to eight people per session; number of sessions or total time period is determined by the organization

Appropriate Audiovisuals: A small slide projector with rear projection screen; two to three hinged display panels no more than 3 feet high; samples of models, products or materials; handout required

Benefits and Limitations: Limited content and very short time frame; same information repeated in a standard format; time for questions

Tips: Practice oral delivery with use of audiovisual materials carefully because time is limited

Presentation for a Poster Display[15]

Note: The poster display format (Fig. 7–2) is becoming popular because of the number of presentations that can be accommodated in a specified time frame and no audiovisual equipment is needed.

Time: Session lasting 1 to 2 hours; discussion time varies by number and type of questions asked

Format: Presenter discusses visual display with people who stop to look; posters lined up next to each other; poster usually attached by pushpins or double-sided fastening material (e.g., Velcro) to a board or other backing material.

Size of Audience: Varies greatly; some people "cruise by" quickly, some just pick up handouts, others stop to read display and discuss topic

Appropriate Audiovisuals: Text, data, artwork, or photos on paper or poster backing or printed on banner; slides and videos not usually allowed, although computer applications can be used; handouts encouraged

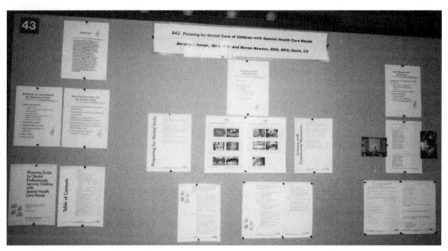

Figure 7–2. Format for poster presentation.

Benefits and Limitations: Opportunity to discuss topic, share ideas, and acquire additional ideas; unpredictable attendance (sometimes crowded and noisy but at other times nobody comes by); not appropriate for topics that require videos or other types of media

Tips: Use color to attract attention and highlight key points; use large, readable print and catchy title; use outline form; intersperse categories of information with charts, graphics, and photos; consider this format for easy setup and transport; include copy of abstract, which is also printed in the program

Presentation for an Oral Paper[16]

Note: The oral paper format usually is part of a session with a theme or a panel.

Time: 10 to 15 minutes, including time for questions

Format: Oral presentation of information (using notes), accompanied by audiovisuals

Size of Audience: Usually more than 30 people but is suitable for hundreds of people

Appropriate Audiovisuals: Slides, overhead transparencies, short videos, computerized presentation

Benefits and Limitations: Large group can be reached; presenter can speak from typed paper or notes; room lighting usually fairly dark; limited interaction with audience; vast array of knowledge in audience

Tips: Try to maintain some eye contact and do not read the paper; use uncomplicated and effective audiovisual materials that highlight important information rather than detract from or repeat information you give orally; practice delivery, timing, and use of audiovisuals before the presentation; decide what information to delete if you are running over time allowance; include transitions between sentences and sections; check audiovisuals and room environment before your session

Presentation for a Round Table Discussion

Note: The round table format (Fig. 7–3) is gaining in popularity for a more informal presentation.

Time: 30 to 60 minutes, presentation sometimes repeated to a new group

Format: Oral presentation and discussion supplemented by audiovisuals to people seated at a round table or in a circle.

Size of Audience: Usually 8 to 10 people

Appropriate Audiovisuals: Handouts, materials, or products, sometimes a short video

Benefits and Limitations: Format allows interactive discussion; participants can introduce themselves and share information with whole table; good for controversial topics or new ideas and programs; limited number of people hear the topic

Tips: Speak from notes or handouts; you will need facilitation skills and ability to refocus group if discussion is off-track or is monopolized by an individual

Figure 7–3. Round table discussion.

Professional presentations can be assessed through the use of course and conference evaluation forms completed by attendees. Evaluation measures usually address the presenter's organization of information, effective use of audiovisuals, relation of theory to practice, knowledge of subject area, and presentation style.

RESOURCES FOR PROFESSIONAL DEVELOPMENT

What avenues are available to dental hygiene students and practitioners to develop skills in health promotion and health presentations? Chapter 6 has outlined the importance of continual review of the scientific literature to keep abreast of new research and trends in dental hygiene research and practice. Because dental public health covers such a broad array of topics, hygienists would benefit by reading literature from other subject areas, such as health education/health promotion, health communications, injury prevention, cancer prevention and early detection, maternal and child health, geriatrics, and school health, to name a few. The many Internet sites devoted to health information facilitate quick perusal of information on any topic and may avoid the limitations of local library systems.

One excellent way to gain experience in actual community settings is through **service-learning programs**. Often referred to as extramural rotations, these programs use structured learning experiences designed by faculty and community member teams in which students provide direct services to groups with identified needs.[17] During the process, students apply concepts learned in the classroom, increasing their understanding of health care systems and community resources. They observe unique community characteristics that affect disease levels, access to care, and delivery of services. In turn, community members learn to appreciate the roles and skills of dental hygienists while receiving needed education and services in their own environment.

Service-learning settings might include day care centers, Head Start programs, public health or migrant health clinics, schools, group homes, residential care facilities, people's own homes, work sites, hospitals, prisons, homeless shelters, adult activity centers, and health departments. Community members serve as adjunct faculty and learning resources. Although faculty members usually arrange these experiences, dental hygiene students may initiate new sites for programs.

Another avenue for updating knowledge, practicing presentation skills, or networking with other professionals is attendance at professional association meetings. Table 7–7 provides an overview of some of the organizations whose missions include the arena of community dental health. Many of these organizations promote student involvement through reduced membership rates and special contests and awards.

Table 7–7

Professional Associations as Resources for Community Dental Health

Organization	Community Oral Health Focus	Publications	Student Membership	Annual Meeting	Office Contacts
American Public Health Associations	Oral Health Section	◆ *Am J Public Health* ◆ *Our Nation's Health* ◆ *Oral Health Section Newsletter*	Yes, $50/yr	Late October, early November	Phone: 202-777-2742 Fax: 202-777-2534 *www.apha.org*
American Association of Public Health Dentistry	Entire focus	◆ *J Public Health Dent* ◆ *Communique Newsletter*	Yes, $35/yr	April or May	Phone: 503-242-0712 Fax: 503-242-0721 *www.aaphd.org*
American Association for Cancer Education	Dental Oncology Section	◆ *J Cancer Educ*	No, membership by nomination	October	Phone: 404-329-7612 Fax: 404-321-4669
Federation of Special Care Organizations in Dentistry: ◆ Academy of Dentistry for Persons with Disabilities ◆ American Association of Hospital Dentists ◆ American Society for Geriatric Dentistry	Selected articles and presentations	◆ *Special Care in Dentistry* ◆ *Newsletter InterFace*	Yes, $33/yr	March or April, Chicago	Phone: 312-440-2660 *www.bgsm.edu/ dentistry/ foscod*
International Federation of Dental Hygienists	Selected articles and presentations	◆ *Contact International*	No, SADHA members qualify, $50/yr	Every 2 years in summer	Sue Lloyd 55 Kemble Rd Forest Hill London SE23 2DH, UK

Table continued on following page

		Table 7-7			
		Professional Associations as Resources for Community Dental Health (*Continued*)			
Organization	**Community Oral Health Focus**	**Publications**	**Student Membership**	**Annual Meeting**	**Office Contacts**
International Association of Dental Research	Scientific groups: ◆ Behavioral Science and Health Services ◆ Geriatric ◆ Oral/Dental Hygiene	◆ *J Dent Res* ◆ *IADR Reports*	Yes, $26/yr	March in North America, every 3rd yr in June or July at international site	Phone: 703-548-0066 Fax: 703-548-1883 *www.iadr.com*
American Dental Education Association	Related sections: ◆ Behavioral Sciences ◆ Community and Preventive Dentistry ◆ Dental	◆ *J Dent Educ* ◆ *Bull Dent Educ*	Yes, $30/yr	March and some regional meetings	Phone: 202-667-9433 *www.aads.jhu. edu*

Summary

We live in a multicultural, global society in which some people are bombarded with health information whereas others are isolated from scientific advances and health information. In the attempt to create a more equitable distribution of resources and information, dental hygienists must broaden their perspectives on how to acquire and provide health information in a credible, appropriate, and effective manner. Ways to accomplish this may include (1) applying well-researched health promotion theories to oral health programs, (2) assessing people's learning styles and information needs, (3) tailoring information in a culturally and linguistically appropriate manner based on needs assessment data, and (4) evaluating the impact of the activities.

Opportunities for using new communication modalities in a variety of settings outside the traditional clinical private practice setting are endless. Service-learning programs and professional associations can be valuable resources for preparing dental hygienists to meet today's health care challenges.

APPLYING YOUR KNOWLEDGE

1. Create a game based on various health promotion theories. You can use the format of well-known games (e.g., Trivial Pursuit, Jeopardy) or a simple matching or fill-in-the-blank format. Students can also work in groups to design role playing scenarios based on the types of behaviors described in the theories.
2. Choose a topic and audience for designing an oral health fact sheet. Describe how you would vary the design and frame the messages according to the following types of communication: (a) generic, (b) targeted, (c) personalized, and (d) tailored.
3. Choose an oral health topic for designing a health promotion activity for consumers (non–health professionals). Each student should select a different audience (e.g., age group, ethnicity) for the materials. The assignment is to (a) describe how you would conduct a needs assessment, (b) select an appropriate educational format, and (c) evaluate the impact of your approach.
4. Choose a topic for a 10-minute presentation. Describe how you would present this topic as (a) a table clinic, (b) a scientific poster, (c) an oral paper, and (d) a round table discussion.
5. Brainstorm ideas for service-learning opportunities, and assume that appropriate resources are available. After the session, check off which ones already are offered to students. Now choose one or two of those not offered and discuss which issues should be considered and which resources would be needed to offer these options. (This activity could lead to a class-initiated project to develop and implement a new service-learning opportunity.)
6. Acquire information, copies of journals and newsletters, and agendas of annual meetings from professional associations, such as those listed in Table 7–7. Compare the organizations for similarities and differences. Students may wish to interview one of the association officers about the history and current involvement of dental hygienists in the organization.

Dental Hygiene Competencies

Reading the material within this chapter and participating in the activities of "Applying Your Knowledge" will contribute to the student's ability to demonstrate the following competencies:

Core Competencies
C.5 Continuously perform self-assessment for lifelong learning and professional growth.
C.8 Communicate effectively with individuals and groups from diverse populations both verbally and in writing.

Community Involvement
CM.4   Facilitate client access to oral health services by influencing individuals and/or organizations for the provisions of oral health care.

Health Promotion
HP.4   Identify individual and population risk factors, and develop strategies that promote health and quality of life.

References

1. Kay E, Locker D: Effectiveness of Oral Health Promotion: A Review. London, Health Education Authority, 1999.
2. Robertson A, Minkler M: New health promotion movement: A critical examination. Health Educ Q 21:295–312, 1994.
3. Glanz K, Rimer BK: Theory at a Glance: A Guide for Health Promotion Practice. Bethesda, Md, National Institutes of Health, 1997.
4. Raczynski JM, DiClemente RJ (eds): Handbook of Health Promotion and Disease Prevention. New York, Kluwer Academic Publishers/Plenum, 1999.
5. An Inventory of Knowledge and Skills Relating to Disease Prevention and Health Promotion. Washington, DC, Association of Teachers of Preventive Medicine, 1994.
6. Wallack L, Dorfman L, Jernigan D, et al: Media Advocacy and Public Health: Power for Prevention. London, Sage Publications, 1993.
7. Kreuter M, Farell D, Olevitch, et al: Tailoring Health Messages: Customizing Communication with Computer Technology. London, Lawrence Erlbaum Associates, 2000.
8. Benn DK, Dankel DD, Clark D, et al: Standardizing data collection and decision-making with an expert system. J Dent Educ 1997; 61:885–894.
9. Bruerd B: Focus groups: Evaluating oral health education materials. Dent Hyg News 1995; 8:21–22.
10. AMC Cancer Research Center: Beyond the Brochure: Alternative Approaches to Effective Health Communication. Atlanta, Centers for Disease Control and Prevention, 1994.
11. DeBiase CB: Dental Health Education: Theory and Practice, 2nd edition. Philadelphia, Lea & Febiger, 1991.
12. DeSouza MB, Kressin NR: Dental health education. In Gluck GM, Morganstein WM: Jong's Community Dental Health, 4th ed. St. Louis, Mosby–Year Book, 1998, pp 177–216.
13. Dignan MB, Carr PA: Program Planning for Health Education and Health Promotion. Philadelphia, Lea & Febiger, 1992.
14. George P. Preparing a table clinic. Dent Hyg News 8:20, 23, 1995.
15. Kelliher GJ, Sachdeva AK: How to present a scientific poster. J Cancer Educ 1996; 11:11–16.
16. Radel J: Effective Presentations. Available from *www.kumc.edu/sait/oted/jradel/effective.html*.
17. Seifer SD, Conners K: A Guide for Developing Community-Responsive Models in Health Professions Education. San Francisco, Community-Campus Partnerships for Health, 1998.

Social Responsibility

Diane Brunson, RDH, MPH

OBJECTIVES

Upon completion of this chapter, the student will be able to:

- Define the terms social responsibility and professional ethics
- Discuss the various opinions surrounding health as a right or a privilege
- Explain how the current delivery of oral health care services affects access
- Identify how the concept of need versus demand affects allocation of resources and the hygienist's role as Consumer Advocate and Educator
- Explain the roles of the dental hygienist as they relate to community education, risk communication, and leadership
- Discuss the responsibility of dental hygienists with respect to cultural competence and their role in providing care to special populations

Key Terms

Social Responsibility	Access	Need
Ethics	Health Security	Demand
Professional Ethics	Pluralistic	Cultural Competence

Opening Statement

Status and Future of Health Care

◆ *The health care system in the United States is in crisis.*

◆ *The public health system in the United States is in disarray.*

◆ *Oral health is a component of overall health, and access to health care services should be a right guaranteed to everyone.*

◆ *Human rights should be the foundation of public health practice, research, and policy in every country in the world.*

◆ *Perceived risks of health care interventions increase when the public receives contradictory opinions from responsible sources.*

▩ SOCIAL RESPONSIBILITY AND PROFESSIONAL ETHICS

Social Responsibility

The following questions are often asked in relation to the responsibilities of the dental hygienist:

- ◆ What are the hygienist's responsibilities to the profession of dental hygiene, to the patients in the dental practice, and to society as a whole?
- ◆ Do these responsibilities entail taking a leadership role in a professional organization?
- ◆ Do they include maintaining competency in clinical skills and currency in dental science so as to provide the best possible care for the patient?
- ◆ Do they look beyond the patients of record in a practice to individuals and communities that lack access to needed oral health care?
- ◆ Do they embrace the art of communication to assure the public that it has the knowledge to improve its own oral health?

Certainly, the responsibilities of the dental hygienist include all of these and more. **Social responsibility** is a broad term that encompasses professionalism, personal and professional ethics, and the role of a profession in the context of the greater society.[1] It includes the concepts of a person's right to health care, the profession's obligation to raise the "dental IQ" of the community, and assuring the health and well-being of the public. In this chapter, by necessity, more questions are asked than answered, but the stage is set for critical thinking and further discussion about individual and collective hygienist's roles, values, and beliefs. The student is encouraged to share thoughts and to discuss personal answers and ideas with colleagues.

Professional Ethics

A term often equated with social responsibility is **ethics,** commonly defined as the general science of right and wrong conduct.[2] Add to this the concept of moral action, and discussions emerge regarding which moral principles should govern a particular action. So intertwined and abstract is this concept that the terms "ethics" and "morals" are often used interchangeably.[3]

Professional ethics, then, is the code by which the profession regulates actions and sets standards for its members, with the recognition that professionals are accountable for their actions.[4] This code serves as a guide to the profession to ensure a high standard of competency, to strengthen the relationships among its members, and to promote the welfare of the entire community.[5] The Code of Ethics of the American Dental Hygienists Association (ADHA) provides this guidance to the dental hygiene profession.

By virtue of the education, the written and clinical board examinations, and subsequent state licensure, dental hygiene is a profession, and dental hygienists are professionals and thus are required to make choices in practice that necessitate ethical decision making. Disagreements occasionally arise from different interpretations of the "proper" roles, responsibilities, and level of decision making of professionals involved in patients' oral care.[6] Often these discussions take precedence over, and are counterproductive to, the larger issues of serving the needs of the public. Examples include whether dental hygienists should be able to (1) determine which teeth would benefit from sealant placement and (2) practice unsupervised in public health settings.

Another set of debates arises in the attempt to define the term *public,* for instance:

◆ Does the word mean only those individuals who seek dental care? Are they the only ones the dental profession has "responsibility" for?
◆ What is the responsibility of the dental hygienist to the broader group of "public," which includes people without access to oral

health care services, culturally diverse populations, and people with special health care needs?

◆ Do people have a right to receive quality dental health care at a cost they can afford?

◆ What is a fair, or just, distribution of limited dental health care resources?

A SYSTEM IN CRISIS

These questions, to which answers are as diverse as populations themselves, point to the need for a broader look at the general health care system in the United States. Many journals and newspapers report that health care in the nation is in a state of "crisis." Although this statement is resounding in many private and public health circles, it is controversial in the face of the technologic advances in medicine and dentistry that have been responsible for improved health standards not only in the United States but also in many countries of the world. Technology has allowed delivery of advanced surgical and cosmetic dental services to one segment of the population even while significant barriers to accessing even preventive and basic restorative care still exist for others.[7]

It is also apparent that the health care crisis has been recognized, reported, discussed, and debated for more than 50 years, with minimal progress made. The Surgeon General's report on oral health specifically quantifies the disparities in oral health status among underserved populations and the barriers many people face in obtaining care.[8] The health professions, including private and public delivery systems, national and state governments, public apathy, and a general lack of social responsibility on the part of society as a whole all have contributed to the failure of each attempt to render health care accessible to everyone. In one form or another, health reforms have been recommended for several decades; however, these have been implemented with little success, and in most cases oral health care services have not been included.

HEALTH CARE: A PRIVILEGE OR A RIGHT?

Health Care as a Privilege

The crux of the debate is the question of whether health care, including oral health care, is a "right" or a "privilege."[9] Who is responsible for "health?" As one ponders these questions, consider the examples in "Guiding Principles" on the next page.

Guiding Principles

Who Has a Right to Health Care?

◆ Should the person who smokes have access to the same level of health care as the nonsmoker?

◆ Should children who are not eligible for Medicaid and who are living in poverty have access to after-hours treatment for ear infections and prescriptions for antibiotics?

◆ Should the senior citizen on a fixed income have equal access to properly fitting dentures?

◆ Should the immigrant female of childbearing age have access to culturally appropriate examinations and treatment?

If any of the answers is "yes," who is responsible for delivering the health care and who is responsible for paying for it? Many would argue that it should not be only private providers offering reduced fees or donating their services. Additional publicly funded programs with acceptable reimbursement rates and dollars sufficient to serve the needs of the population are also needed. The following questions relate to whose responsibility it is to provide health care services and to pay for them:

◆ Should taxes be increased to support these programs or incentives implemented to increase provider participation?
◆ What is the responsibility of the patient seeking care?
◆ Should access to health care be a privilege of productive members of society who have the ability to pay for that health care?
◆ Are rights automatic, or are they "earned" as a reward for being socially responsible?

These questions have no clear answers, and they challenge the individual provider's values and sense of social responsibility.

Health Care as a Right

The United States Constitution does not specifically guarantee a "right to health," since "health" is a dynamic, continually changing state, unique to each individual.[10] One interpretation is that health and access to health care are not so much a legal right; rather, they are a "moral" right and, as such, are the obligation of society as a whole is to provide care in response to that right, with providers playing an important role.[2] Society, however, has not universally accepted that responsibility despite several key events that have attempted to highlight the relationship between individual rights, human dignity, and the human condition.[11]

In 1946, the Constitution of the World Health Organization (WHO) defined health as "a state of complete physical, mental, and social well-being" (see Chapter 1). This was reiterated in the Universal Declaration of Human Rights adopted by the United Nations General Assembly on December 10, 1948 (Article 25):

> Everyone has the right to a standard of living adequate for the health and well-being of himself and of his family, including food, clothing, housing and medical care. . . .[12]

An amendment to the Public Health Service Act, passed by Congress in 1966, states that "promoting and assuring the highest level of health attainable for every person serves the nation's best interests."

The fundamental basis of human rights is the recognition of the equal worth and dignity of everyone and implies that individuals, institutions, and society as a whole should protect and promote health and should ensure that health is neither impaired nor at risk. When the health of people has been left solely to the current health services system, many population groups have been left without access to health care and with little or no constituency advocating for their right to that care. Increasingly, this system has not been able to keep pace with the number of uninsured patients, expanding populations, shifts in demographics, degradation of the environment, and changes in lifestyles and value systems. This discussion becomes pertinent in the field of dental public health, which focuses on the prevention of oral diseases and promotes population-based health activities to ensure the oral health of all people.

ACCESS TO ORAL HEALTH CARE

It is essential to understand the term **access** and its relationship to social responsibility. Access is assuring that conditions are in place for people to obtain the care they need and want.[13] The key word here is "assuring." Many lawmakers and health providers feel that their responsibility is not *to provide* but to make sure that services *are provided* through different means and combinations with other partners. Herrell and Mulholland have termed this latter form of assurance **health security.**[14]

The World Health Organization further defines health security in terms of "the rights and conditions that enable individuals to attain and enjoy their full potential for a healthy life." However, some practitioners and lawmakers do not want the obligation of providing universal and comprehensive health services and do not want any resemblance to "socialized medicine," a system in which the means of funding and distributing health care is centralized, usually with a government entity.

As a result, in the United States a **pluralistic** system has evolved in which numerous, distinct health care delivery systems coexist simultaneously.[9] In dentistry, this translates to private offices, community health centers, Medicaid-only and nonprofit clinics, mobile vans, school-based health centers, and hospital clinics and emergency departments, each with set criteria determining which patients will receive services according to socioeconomic, geographic, age, and cultural variables. In some cases, this pluralistic system works well, but it is also easy to see how many populations are confused by the complexity of the system, thus "falling through the cracks" and not receiving any dental services.

DISTRIBUTION OF HEALTH RESOURCES

Shortage of Dental Professionals

The result of the health services system's inability to keep pace with a rapidly changing society is a maldistribution—and, in some instances, a "shortage"—of health care providers; such conditions have a direct impact on access to services. Many might convincingly argue that there has been a shortage of dental hygienists in the 1990s and predict an even greater shortage of dentists and hygienists by the year 2010.

However, the shortage is a complicated phenomenon. It includes the closure of several dental and dental hygiene schools in the last several years, the varied length of time dental professionals remain in clinical practice, and part-time versus full-time employment opportunities. The shortage is particularly evident in the fields of dental education and dental public health, where salaries and benefits have not kept pace with those available in private practice settings.[15] Finally, insufficient numbers of culturally diverse dental professionals are trained and are entering the work force to provide care to underserved populations.

Need versus Demand

With the ratio of providers to population decreasing, who determines who receives what level of services? The concept of "need versus demand" enters the discussion. Briefly defined, **need** refers to those services deemed by the health professional to be necessary after a variety of assessment and diagnostic tools, and perhaps past experience, have been employed. **Demand** refers to the health care services desired by the individual or community. The dental profession is partly driven by society's perception of what is acceptable and unacceptable in terms of health and aesthetics (e.g., bleaching); consequently, need and demand are sometimes in close approximation.

When tremendous differences exist between need and demand in a community, however, it is imperative that health care providers educate the public and policymakers regarding what is needed to bring public demand as close to what is needed as possible for optimal use of scarce resources. Herein lies a major social responsibility of dental hygienists and other health care providers: education and communication.

As an example, in state Children with Special Health Care Needs (CSHCN) programs, limited funding is available for orthodontic services for low-income children with severe malocclusions. The qualifying malocclusions are usually due to skeletal malformations, resulting in impaired speech and chewing ability, and to facial asymmetry (as in cleft lip and palate) and are not due simply to an overbite or overjet, malalignment of several teeth, or cross-bite. The difference is often difficult for families desiring aesthetically appealing smiles for their children to understand why funds are going to other children for the restoration of functional occlusion. Educating families of children, public health providers, and lawmakers becomes as important as paying for needed services.

An important component and a useful tool in reconciling need and demand is the use of *dental indices* (see Chapter 4). Using Dean's Fluorosis Index, the Community Periodontal Index (CPI), the Decayed, Missing, and Filled Teeth (DMFT) Index, and the WHO Dental Aesthetic Index (DAI) gives health care professionals objective data to use when communicating to policymakers and individuals about the oral health care needs in their community and provides the basis for decisions.

PATIENT RESPONSIBILITY

An earlier question in this chapter concerned the patient's role in accessing health care. In a society where a pluralistic health system exists, greater emphasis is placed on individual responsibility for health; however, when we look at the significant advances in any nation's health to date, personal lifestyle has not been the most important factor.[16] This is particularly true for improvements in overall oral health status, which can certainly be attributed to community water fluoridation, fluoride toothpaste, sealants, and better restorative materials.

Three factors have been associated with health care inequalities and increased burden of disease: (1) education, (2) housing, and (3) nutrition. Each of these factors is recognized by society as primarily the responsibility of government and publicly funded programs.[16] Those in favor of multiple oral health service delivery systems claim that increased patient responsibility would reduce the "demand" for oral health services. This would be easier than manipulating the way in which oral health services are provided, thereby helping to resolve the health care access dilemma.[17] Although prevention would go a long way toward reducing the need for emergency and episodic care, when we consider the 10 greatest public health achievements of the 20th century (see Chapter 1), very little individual patient responsibility was involved. Some historians point out that most of these significant advances occurred during that century's "infectious disease" era; in today's "information age," however, perhaps increased personal responsibility is appropriate.

Particularly difficult is assigning personal responsibility to children whose dental caries experience, for example, reflects the socioeconomic and educational constraints of their parents and caregivers; or to the elderly, who experience increased periodontal disease, decay, incidence of oral cancer, and tooth loss as income becomes fixed or decreases. Some believe that this type of health status data provides an important indicator of the degree to which human rights are enjoyed or denied as a result of inequity and discrimination. The inequality comes around full circle as declines in dental health and overall health perpetuate the inability to improve socioeconomic status.

This is not to say that individuals should not have responsibility for improving their own oral health, participating in conscientious brushing, flossing, and regular dental visits. According to the results of the Behavioral Risk Factor Surveillance Survey (BRFSS), the primary response adults give for not seeing a dentist in the past year is that they "did not see a reason to go." The dental hygienist, in the role of Educator and Consumer advocate, is in an ideal position to communicate the importance of regular oral health care and the relationship to general health and systemic disease, not only to patients but to the public as a whole.

▨ RISK COMMUNICATION

Understanding Risk

Another aspect of social and professional responsibility is communication. Not only are health education, oral hygiene instruction, and post-treatment instructions and follow-up of paramount importance; so is the communication of "risk." It is the responsibility of the dental profession, including dental hygienists, to know what the public perceives as risk and to be able to assist in bringing to light peer-reviewed research to reduce public misperceptions.

For example, a segment of the general public perceives inherent risks in radiographs, amalgam restorations, biofilms in dental unit water lines, instrument sterilization techniques, transmission of disease (e.g., human immunodeficiency virus infection, hepatitis) in dental offices, and fluoridation of community water supplies. It is the dental hygienist's responsibility to become knowledgeable about current research regarding these issues for ensuring compliance with recommended protocols, regardless of the practice setting, to minimize these risks. The next task is to communicate pertinent information to the public in order to reduce the spread of misinformation.

Communication

The messages obtained by the public regarding oral health issues are judged, primarily, not on their content but on whether the person providing the information is someone who inspires trust.[17] As a group, dentists and hygienists are regarded as very trustworthy, but this trust is understandably shaken when a member of the profession openly opposes water fluoridation, advocates removing amalgam fillings for reasons other than recurrent decay or fracture, or blatantly dismisses current infection control guidelines.

Communication is a two-way process, and to fully understand a community's concerns, the professional responsible for communicating risk must take these concerns seriously while providing sound scientific evidence. This is where the hygienist's role in staying abreast of current research and utilizing skills in critically evaluating scientific research and literature not only is important but also is a component of the profession's social responsibility.

Comparative Analysis

Communicating risk is not an easy task. Many professionals use "comparative" risk analyses, which are not always effective and may be a hindrance in conveying trust.[17] Following are a few examples of potential risks in dentistry:

1. For the patient concerned about a full set of radiographs, x-ray exposure is explained as being comparable to 1 hour out in the sun at high altitude.
2. For the patient hesitant to accept amalgam fillings as part of a treatment plan because of the mercury content, the mercury level is considered comparable to that in common foods.
3. For the community resident fearful of 1 part per million (ppm) of fluoride in the water supply, the amount is said to be comparable to one drop of water in a bathtub half full.

Providing these comparisons is not necessarily incorrect, but whether such information can succeed in allaying the concerns of the individual is unpredictable. Herein lies another key point: Scientist and professional tend to define "risk" in terms of entire populations; laypeople are concerned with the risk to themselves. Each person approaches risk from different frames of reference based on past experience, culture, and the media.

Perceived Risk

In addition to the problems of comparisons, according to Peter Bennett, are "fright factors."[18] Popular antifluoridation arguments and the perceived risks based on these fright factors are outlined in Table 8–1.

Antifluoridation arguments include claims that the presence of fluoride in community water makes consumption of fluoride "involuntary and inescapable" and that some "at-risk" individuals have adverse reactions to fluoride (e.g., allergies, cancer), which remain unsubstantiated; however,

	Table 8–1	
	Perceived Fluoridation Risks	
Factors That Heighten Perceived Risk		**Popular Antifluoridation Arguments to Illustrate Perceived Risk**
1. Exposure is involuntary versus voluntary.		1. Fluoride in community drinking water is unavoidable.
2. Risk is unevenly distributed (some people have problems; others do not).		2. People with suppressed immune systems may be adversely affected by fluoride.
3. Risk is inescapable despite personal precaution.		3. Fluoride is in nearly all foods and beverages.
4. Source is unfamiliar.		4. Fluoride chemicals are a by-product of fertilizer industry.
5. Fluoride is man-made rather than natural.		5. Chemicals used in the process include sodium fluoride, which is different from the calcium fluoride occurring in nature.
6. Hidden and irreversible damage may result.		6. Overexposure in the young results in fluorosis in permanent teeth.
7. Particular danger may be posed to children or pregnant women.		7. Warning on toothpaste tube cautions against swallowing the paste.
8. Illness, injury, or death is possible.		8. Chronic overexposure may result in crippling skeletal fluorosis.
9. Damage occurs to real people, not anonymous victims.		9. Fluoridated water is not used in kidney dialysis because of possible overdosing of fluoride, resulting in death.
10. Fluoridation is poorly understood by science.		10. Caries have decreased in nonfluoridated communities.
11. Statements from responsible sources have been contradictory.		11. Some health professions are opposed to fluoridation.

adding to the difficulty is the fact that some arguments against fluoridation are true. For instance, fluoride chemicals are a by-product of the fertilizer industry, there is a printed warning on fluoride toothpaste tubes about not swallowing the paste, and the prevalence of dental caries is declining in nonfluoridated communities. However, these statements are used inappropriately and incorrectly when one is discussing fluoridating community water supplies at optimal levels.

The public does not always understand the differences. It is evident why some perceived risks, such as fluoridation, trigger so many more alarms than other health interventions regardless of the scientific basis or evidence to the contrary. The right column of Table 8–1 can easily be changed from "fluoridation" to "amalgam" for another illustration of why perceived risk is a communication challenge.

Responsibility in Communication

Risks not only are dependent on the context in which they are presented but also are intertwined with personal values; thus, it becomes difficult to dismiss the antifluoridation arguments as "unreasonable." Attitudes about certain risks are often influenced by how people believe society should be; their relationship with nature; the benefits and disadvantages of technology; cultural influences; and, occasionally, religious beliefs.

Successful risk communication raises the level of people's understanding of relevant issues and reassures those involved that they are adequately informed within the limits of available knowledge.[19] It is a social responsibility of the dental professional to communicate risk. Successful communication is dependent on respecting beliefs, gathering information consistent with the public's point of view, and then providing a professional account of the evidence underlying sound health decisions and treatment modalities.

SPECIAL POPULATIONS

Cultural Sensitivity

A brief discussion of "special populations" and society's responsibility in ensuring their access to health care is warranted. Special populations include:

- Low-income patients (Medicaid recipients, the working poor, homeless people)
- Patients of various cultures (farm workers, immigrants, Native Americans) who may have different life experiences and backgrounds as well as language barriers
- Patients who are immunocompromised (those with human immunodeficiency virus [HIV] infection/acquired immunodeficiency syndrome [AIDS] and those undergoing chemotherapy or radiation therapy for cancer)
- Women and children in shelters
- Troubled teens
- Nursing home residents
- Patients with Alzheimer's disease
- Mentally and physically disabled persons

Often the traditional dental office setting does not match the needs of the special-population patient. Case managers, social workers, and school nurses are commonly expected to provide education to these populations on how to access the dental office. Look around a dental office or dental hygiene school clinic, and observe how it might welcome a special population patient. For example:

- Would a Medicaid patient feel comfortable in the waiting room?
- Are written materials, health histories, informed consents, and post-operative instructions translated into other languages and at a literacy level appropriate for the community?
- Is the office or clinic located on a major public transportation route?
- Has someone arranged for a translator (other than a patient's family member) to help the patient understand the diagnosis, treatment, and follow-up instructions?
- Would the people be better served by bringing the dental clinic to them?
- Is the dental staff culturally diverse?

Cultural Competence

These aforementioned considerations fall in the category of **cultural competence** and affect the profession's responsibility in reducing the burden (incidence) of disease. Special populations typically have a higher burden of oral disease and face many barriers to accessing care.[20]

For example, community health centers often employ bilingual or bicultural staff members to encourage access by minority populations. Many populations respond more favorably to health messages from someone of their own culture and language. Health centers serving farm worker populations often have mobile vans that go directly into the fields to provide health education, take blood pressure readings, conduct oral health screenings, and give vaccinations. Patients scheduled for a follow-up appointment are more likely to keep the appointment if someone has reached out to them in a culturally sensitive manner.

Mobile vans and portable equipment also serve low-income populations, as in school-based sealant programs; and mentally and physically disabled persons are served through the National Foundation of Dentistry for the Handicapped's Homebound Dentistry Programs. Native American populations, many served through the Indian Health Service (IHS), often have clinics of their own design and controlled by tribal councils, utilizing IHS or contract providers.

Alternative Practice Settings

In states where dental hygienists are allowed to practice under general supervision or allowed to practice unsupervised in public health settings, many hygienists have found rewarding careers providing preventive services using portable equipment in long-term care facilities. Some facilities have set aside rooms with a full dental operatory to make it easier for residents to seek care.

Many states that have school-based health centers (SBHCs) are beginning to research the feasibility of adding dental services to their centers. A few have implemented full dental clinics with paid and volunteer dentists and hygienists, whereas others contract with public and private entities with portable equipment to provide preventive and restorative services. Military personnel (e.g., the National Guard) have also set up portable units in rural and inner city areas to provide dental care closer to home for underserved populations. Still other communities use state-of-the-art mobile dental clinics to reach rural and frontier areas and special populations.

All of these examples illustrate sensitivity to the increasing cultural diversity of communities and address the needs of special populations by assuring access to oral health services. Many of these alternative dental delivery systems rely on volunteers and donated services because of limited funding and competing community priorities. By bringing the services *to* special populations in a manner consistent with and comfortable to their culture, dental professionals have been able to provide increased access to services and have helped to improve oral health as well as general health.[21]

▨ PATIENT CONFIDENTIALITY

In addition to the dental professional's responsibilities in respecting cultures, maintaining patient confidentiality is paramount. The rights of the patient and maintaining patient confidentiality in private practice settings are emphasized throughout the dental hygiene student's clinical education; however, it is often forgotten that the same principles apply in dental public health practice.

In public health settings, which may include clinics, schools, and health fair screenings, the atmosphere is often less structured and more chaotic at times, thus necessitating greater attention to patient confidentiality. Ensuring a patient's right to privacy during screenings and treatment, protecting records (signed consents and medical histories), and refraining from sharing personal patient information (e.g., HIV status) with school personnel, policymakers, and other patients are part of the social and ethical responsibilities of the dental professional.

Community groups commonly desire to highlight their successful projects by inviting media from newspapers and television to showcase their efforts. However, it is prudent to gain permission from patients if they are going to be in any photographs or film coverage. Many schools require signed permission forms from parents if their child is to be photographed. Inclusion of as many partners in the community as possible in the planning process helps to avoid these social mishaps and ensures program visibility and success.

▨ CHILD ABUSE AND NEGLECT

In the dental hygienist's role in helping to promote the health and well-being of the public, difficult situations sometimes arise that test social and ethical principles and values. In many states, the dental hygienist is a mandated reporter of suspected child abuse and neglect. This means that the hygienist is required by law to report to the appropriate authorities any information regarding a child whom the hygienist suspects is a victim of abuse or neglect. PANDA (Prevent Abuse and Neglect through Dental Awareness) programs provide training to dental professionals on recognizing and reporting suspected cases of child abuse and neglect, including dental neglect.[22]

As a mandated reporter, the dental hygienist should be alert for these signs of abuse:

- Bruises, particularly around the areas of the head and neck
- Bruises of various colors, which indicate multiple stages of healing
- Injuries inconsistent with stories of how they occurred
- Inappropriate clothing for the temperature (long-sleeved sweaters in hot, humid climates)
- Unusual shyness or withdrawal or a reaction to oral procedures

These signs should raise questions as to whether abuse may have occurred. Parental disregard of or refusal to follow through on a child's needed dental treatment may be an indication of dental neglect. It is the professional responsibility of hygienists to know the legal requirements in the community, the agency to call in order to report gathered information, and the steps to take to ensure safety for themselves as well as for the patient.

LEADERSHIP

For every child without medical insurance, 2.6 children are without dental insurance; and for every adult with medical insurance, 3 adults are without dental insurance.[8] With the increasing number of people without health or dental insurance, continued leadership on the part of dental professionals to eliminate oral health disparities and to assure access to oral health services for all is needed.

Dental hygiene leadership embraces the following concepts:

- Social responsibility
- Professionalism
- Ethics
- Communication
- Cultural competence (see earlier)

A leader in dental hygiene works within the community to develop consensus on what "oral health care for all" might look like. He or she enables others to see the problem at first hand and to implement solutions and models public health practice by assuring equal access to care and not tolerating discrimination against any person seeking care. The leader encourages other professionals in the community to participate in health promotion and disease prevention activities and celebrates successes.

The dental hygiene leader challenges "the way things have always been done" and seeks new ways to maximize resources and productivity while remaining mindful of ethical decision-making processes and commitment to quality oral care.[23] The leader respects the other health care providers in the community and forges collaborative relationships in providing total health care for the public.

Finally, the dental hygiene leader works within the profession to ensure continued competency, lifelong learning, and maintenance of quality standards of practice.

Summary

The dental hygienist is a professional. Inherent in the role of the professional is the responsibility of making ethical decisions and choices and opportunities to practice dental hygiene in ways that will increase access to oral health services for all populations. The role requires the leadership to uphold the standards of dental hygiene practice and communication skills to promote optimal oral health for all.

APPLYING YOUR KNOWLEDGE

1. Conduct a survey of other students on campus, or dental professionals in the community, as to their beliefs of access to health care as a "privilege" or a "right." Present your findings to your class, allowing time for discussion of the various views collected.
2. Choose a dental treatment or preventive measure that is perceived by some members of society as carrying risk. Research two scientific articles in response to one of those perceived risks, and share your expertise with the rest of your class.
3. Invite oral health care professionals in the community who provide services to special populations as the majority of the practice to participate in a panel discussion describing the following:
   a. What they see in terms of the burden of disease among their patients
   b. How they view their role in improving access to care
   c. What they view as their responsibility to the public at large
4. Visit an alternative dental services delivery system (mobile, portable, long-term care, school-based health center), and observe whether the system improves access to oral health services for a special population.

Create a poster that compares and contrasts this system with the traditional dental office in terms of:

a. Access for that population
b. Dental services provided
c. Cost per patient
d. Utilization of auxiliaries

5. Consider the following community situation involving social responsibility:

Jan has been volunteering in a second-grade school-based sealant project, operated by the local health department at several elementary schools in the city. Volunteer dentists screen the children to ascertain which teeth are sealable and to prioritize children for urgency of restorative needs. The dental hygienists then apply sealant to the approved teeth, provide one-on-one oral hygiene instruction, and work with school nurses to provide case management and follow-up for restorative needs. One particular child, Joey, has six decayed primary teeth. He is irritable and fearful in the dental chair. Because he is not a legal citizen, Joey does not have insurance and is not eligible for Medicaid.

Upon preparing to place the sealants, Jan notices that teeth Nos. 3, 19, and 30 are approved for sealants. Tooth No. 14 is checked as needing a restoration; however, it is evident to Jan that tooth No. 3 needs the restoration and tooth No. 14 is perhaps sealable, suggesting that the teeth numbers have been switched at screening. Jan does not seal the upper molars until the tooth numbers can be clarified, and she seals the lower molars. She sends a follow-up note home to Joey's parents indicating the findings of the screening and the urgent need for dental care.

Jan returns to the school 3 months later to conduct a sealant retention check on the children who had received sealants. She discovers that (1) the status of teeth Nos. 3 and 14 for sealants has not been clarified and (2) Joey has not received the urgent dental treatment. Upon talking with the school nurse, Jan finds that the screening dentist has not been back to re-screen and that the nurse has been unsuccessful in convincing Joey's mother to take him to the dentist and has not found any local dental providers willing to donate the needed dental services.

1. What should Jan have done regarding the apparent switch in teeth numbers for sealants?

a. Do as she did; do not seal either one, and wait for a rescreening by the dentist.

b. Note the apparent switch in the child's chart, and seal tooth No. 14.

c. Call the screening dentist, and explain the situation in order to try to get verbal approval to seal tooth No. 14.

d. Indicate in the chart that tooth No. 3 is not sealable, and leave both teeth Nos. 3 and 14 for restorations.

2. What is Jan's responsibility concerning Joey's urgent need for dental care?

   a. She does not have any responsibility. It is up to the child's parents to get him into the dentist.

   b. She needs to work with the school nurse to find dental care for Joey as soon as possible.

   c. She needs to call Social Services to report a suspected case of dental neglect.

   d. She needs to talk to Joey's mother to explain the urgency of the situation.

3. What is Jan's responsibility to the dental professional community at large, in that the school nurse has not been able to find anyone to take Joey?

   a. She does not have any responsibility because dentists can decide whom they want in their practices.

   b. She should file a complaint with the state dental licensing board.

   c. She should make a presentation to local dentists regarding the oral health status of the children and their unmet dental needs.

   d. She should follow the dental professional's lead and try to convince Joey's parents that his dental needs are a priority and that they need to find the resources to pay for it.

1. c. It is doubtful that Joey will be getting the restorative care he needs in the next few days; he is in the chair waiting for sealants, which will provide him with a much-needed preventive measure. A phone call to the screening dentist would probably resolve the discrepancy, with a verbal referral to the hygienist's judgment, and the correct tooth can be sealed.

2. b. Although it is often tempting to jump in and try to talk directly with parents in school settings to ensure that dental care is received, the hygienist can quickly become overwhelmed with these case management details. It is more cost-effective to work with the school nurse, who knows the families; to identify the barriers to Joey's family seeking care; to provide suggestions to the nurse regarding potential resources; and to follow up weekly to make sure that treatment has been arranged.

3. c. Local dental providers are reluctant to take on too many uninsured patients because they become overwhelmed very quickly, since they become known in the community as taking the uninsured. However, many dentists do take case-by-case referrals, once they are informed of the needs in the community, and they often work together to set up a system for sharing the burden of these difficult cases. In this instance, it is the hygienist's responsibility to share with the dental community, and all other interested parties in the community, the oral health needs of the children so that solutions to providing needed dental care can be implemented and resources obtained.

Dental Hygiene Competencies

Reading the material in this chapter and participating in the activities of "Applying Your Knowledge" will contribute to the student's ability to demonstrate the following competencies:

Core Competencies
C.1   Apply a professional code of ethics in all endeavors.
C.6   Advance the profession through service activities and affiliations with professional organizations.
C.8   Communicate effectively with individuals and groups from diverse populations, both verbally and in writing.

Health Promotion and Disease Prevention
HP.1   Promote the values of oral and general health and wellness to the public and organizations within and outside the profession.

Community Involvement
CM.4   Facilitate client access to oral health care services by influencing individuals and organizations for the provision of oral health care.

References

1. Woolfolk MW: The social responsibility model. J Dent Educ 57(5):346–348, 1993.
2. Ozar DT, Love J: Conflicting values in oral health care. J Am Coll Dent 65(3):15–18, 1998.
3. Ozar DT, Sokol DJ: Dental Ethics at Chairside: Professional Principles and Practical Application. St. Louis, Mosby–Year Book, 1994.
4. Gaston MA: Survey of ethical issues in dental hygiene. J Dent Hyg 64(5):217–24, 1990.
5. Frankel MS: Taking ethics seriously: Building a professional community. J Dent Hyg 66(9):386–392, 1992.
6. Weinstein BD: Dental Ethics. Philadelphia, Lea & Febiger, 1993.
7. Gershen JA: Response to the social responsibility model: The convergence of curriculum and health policy. J Dent Educ 57(5):350–352, 1993.
8. Oral Health in America: A Report of the Surgeon General—Executive Summary. Rockville, Md, U.S. Department of Health and Human Services, National Institute of Dental and Craniofacial Research (NIDCR), National Institutes of Health, 2000.
9. Stewart GT: Health care in America: Privilege or right? Lancet 2(7737):1305–1306, 1971.
10. Burt BA, Eklund SA: Dentistry, Dental Practice, and the Community, 4th ed. Philadelphia, WB Saunders, 1992.
11. Goldsmith MF: Health and human rights inseparable. JAMA 270(5):553, 1993.
12. United Nations: Universal declaration of human rights. Available at *http://www.unhchr.ch/udhr/lang/eng.htm.*
13. Isman R, Isman B: Oral Health America White Paper: Access to Oral Health Services in the U.S. 1997 and Beyond. Funding from the Robert Wood Johnson Foundation, 1997.
14. Herrel IC, Mulholland CA: Reflections on health in development and human rights. World Health Stat Q 51(1):88–92, 1998.
15. Valacovitch R: Dental education and emerging trends: Challenges for U.S. dental schools. American Academy of Dental Schools, Executive Director's Report to the Legislative Advisory Committee, 2000.
16. Sarll DW: Who is responsible for good oral health? Br Dent J 180(5):164–167, 1996.

17. Bent JP: Health access and social responsibility. Arch Otolaryngol Head Neck Surg 118(3):344, 1992.
18. Bennett P, Calman K: Risk Communication and Public Health. Oxford, UK, University of Oxford Press, 1999.
19. Deahl ST II, Kromer ME: A taxonomy for lay risk perceptions of dentistry. J Public Health Dent 56(4):213–218, 1996.
20. Warren RC: Oral Health for All: Policy for Available, Accessible, and Acceptable Care. Washington DC, Center for Policy Alternatives, 1999.
21. Jenny J: Basic social values, structural elements in oral health systems and oral health status. Int Dent J 30(3):276–285, 1980.
22. American Academy of Pediatrics/American Academy of Pediatric Dentistry: Oral and dental aspects of child abuse and neglect: Joint statement. Pediatrics 104(2):348–350, 1999.
23. Kouzes JM, Posner BZ: The Leadership Challenge. San Francisco, Jossey-Bass, 1995.

Test-Taking Strategies and Community Cases

Kathy Voigt Geurink, RDH, MA

OBJECTIVES

Upon completion of this chapter, the student will be able to:

◆ Develop an overview of the National Board Dental Hygiene Examination

◆ Develop guidelines for answering multiple-choice test items and community testlets

◆ Identify tips for examination preparation

◆ Take a practice examination on community cases

◆ Increase his or her confidence level in preparing for the examination

Community Health Activities	Multiple-Choice Questions Community Cases	Critical Thinking

OVERVIEW OF THE EXAMINATION

The National Board Dental Hygiene Examination (NBDHE) is written and administered by the Joint Commission on National Dental Examinations of the American Dental Association. The purpose of the examination is to determine professional competency in the various subject areas that are taught in the schools of dental hygiene.

According to the NBDHE Candidate Guide, the examination consists of 350 multiple-choice questions and is administered during 1 full day consisting of two 4-hour periods. Component A (4 hours in the morning) contains approximately 200 multiple-choice questions; Component B (4 hours in the afternoon) contains 150 questions based on 12 to 15 dental hygiene cases. Component A is composed of the following three major areas:

- Scientific basis for dental hygiene practice
- Provision of clinical dental hygiene services
- **Community health activities**

In the community health activities area, approximately four **community cases** are presented with a series of **multiple-choice questions** related to the situation described. The community cases are simulated situations that might occur in the community. They usually involve the dental hygienist's participation in a community oral health activity. Multiple-choice questions following the community cases require that the dental hygiene student apply information, such as that within this textbook, to select the correct answer. The community cases and the related questions are referred to as *testlets* within the examination.

MULTIPLE-CHOICE QUESTIONS

Multiple-choice questions are used to test the student's knowledge and understanding of content. A multiple-choice test item consists of a *stem*, which poses a problem that is followed by a list of answers. The stem is presented either as a question or as an incomplete statement. A choice of four or five answers is given per question. Only one of the answers is correct or best. The other answers are called *distractors*. Following are some suggestions:

1. When answering multiple test questions, use your time wisely. Look over the test initially to determine how many questions are presented, and calculate approximately how much time you will need to answer them.

2. Read directions and questions carefully.
3. Attempt to answer every question; if you are unsure of an answer, mark that question to enable you to return to it later if time permits.
4. Actively reason through each question, and read all the answers before making your choice.

Here are some tips that may help you in answering the questions. Look for the following within the questions and answers:

* Logical clues that help you select the correct answer
* A repeated word or concept in both the question and answer
* Length of the correct response: often the longest answer
* A similarity in or a direct opposite of responses; you can eliminate contradictory answers or complete opposites to the question

Examples of Multiple-Choice Questions

The following multiple-choice test questions relate to information in Chapter 7 and demonstrate how to answer multiple-choice questions using the clues already presented. Answer the following questions using your knowledge and these clues.

1. Which choice describes the Stages of Change Theory?
   a. It is an example of ways to effect changes in public policy
   b. It assesses a person's readiness to change and adopt behaviors that lead to a healthy lifestyle
   c. It includes key concepts such as reciprocal determination, observational learning, and reinforcement
   d. It directly assesses how susceptible a patient perceives oneself to be to periodontitis

2. An example of the tailoring technique that is used in formulating an individual's oral health plan is:
   a. Highlighting one or two messages that might apply to your patient
   b. Using photographs of American Indian women for posters in the Indian Health Service clinic
   c. Providing three individualized recommendations based on risk factors identified during a personal risk assessment
   d. Asking a group whether they prefer a video, slides, or a demonstration

3. You have developed a new program to promote oral health to teenaged mothers. You would like to discuss your ideas with other health professionals at an upcoming public health conference. Which of the following formats would be best for presenting your information?
   a. Round table discussion
   b. Oral presentation

    c. Research poster presentation

    d. Table clinic

4. Which of the following formats would you use to ensure the highest retention of information about oral cancer in a group of adults?

    a. Reading a booklet about oral cancer

    b. Using a multimedia presentation

    c. Demonstrating an oral examination, followed by a discussion and a return demonstration of how to perform the oral cancer examination

    d. Watching a video

The answers to these questions are provided here using clues versus a knowledge rationale. See Chapter 7 for a knowledge review.

1. b. This is the *logical* answer because Chapter 7 is on health promotion and behavioral change. Although a. has the word *change,* the topic is not relevant. Answers c. and d. have no wording similar to that of the question.

2. c. This answer uses a *similar* idea—the concept of individualization—even if one does not connect risk with tailoring. Answers b. and d. can be eliminated because they are opposites of the question, referring to groups rather than an individual. Answer a. uses the vague term *might*, which makes it a less viable answer than c.

3. a. This answer uses *repetition* of the term *discuss*, which gives the clue to the best answer. The other three answers are ways to present the information, but a. is the best answer.

4. c. This answer has *length*, and it is logical that you will retain information better when you involve more of your senses.

▨ ANSWERING COMMUNITY CASE QUESTIONS

When answering the community cases, you must change your train of thought from thinking about private practice to thinking community. Recall the definitions from within this text and the comparisons of private practice and community oral health practice. Your selection of the correct answer must be in relation to what is best for the community as a whole. You will be applying the information you have learned in your community course to a simulated situation in the community.

    In most dental hygiene schools, students have an opportunity to apply the information that they have learned in the community course by conducting projects in the community. These projects require **critical thinking** skills to determine the best way to achieve maximum oral health for the population the student chooses to work with. Studying the "Applying

Your Knowledge" features at the end of each chapter in this textbook is a good way for students to practice their critical thinking skills. Testing with cases requires students not only to retrieve knowledge, as in the stand-alone multiple-choice questions, but also to use their knowledge and critical thinking skills to make choices. Your critical thinking skills are just that—thinking about what you know. The NBDHE measures your ability to solve problems and to make decisions based on the knowledge you have acquired in your course work.

Once you are in a community frame of mind, read carefully through the community situation. Then start on the multiple-choice questions; remember that the questions refer to the case presented. Some of the questions can probably be answered on a stand-alone basis, but they are intended to relate only to the case presented. The best answer is the one related to the information in the case.

If time permits, rereading through the case one more time after answering the questions allows you to catch any incorrect answer you may have selected without recalling important information from within the case. The community cases are located in the test in the latter half of the morning. If you do better with case-type questions early in a 4-hour period, consider answering the cases first and then the other multiple-choice questions in this section.

In your general preparation for the examination, try to identify your weak areas and concentrate your review on them. Do not cram for an examination of this magnitude. Set aside scheduled time for review, possibly using a calendar to set aside hours weekly to use for study. Some people study well in groups. Group studying can be beneficial because you learn other students' ideas and ways to recall information. Other students do better alone. It is your choice, but perhaps you can try a little of both.

Previous examination questions give you practice in test taking and often cover material that never changes. Alternate your review periods with practice examinations. Staying calm is important to your psyche. Remember, you won't know everything. A positive attitude always helps!

▨ EXAMPLES OF CRITICAL THINKING: COMMUNITY ORAL HEALTH PRACTICE TESTLETS

The following four testlets and community cases are compiled as a practice test in community oral health. The number and type of questions are similar to what you will encounter on the NBDHE in this area. You should complete these questions in less than 40 minutes so that you will still have about 1 minute per question on the other multiple-choice questions in the morning section. There are four testlets with five questions each.

TESTLET NO. 1

You practice dental hygiene in a low-socioeconomic-level, multicultural city with a population of 1.5 million. The office you work in, however, serves a relatively higher socioeconomic population of the city. The city water supply is not fluoridated; consequently, dental decay is prevalent in the mouths of children residing in the poorer sections of the city. The majority of families in the city are of Hispanic descent. You recently assisted the public health dental hygienist in conducting a screening on the children in a local elementary school to document their oral health status. Fluoridation was defeated 10 years ago because of a strong antifluoridation campaign. Fluoridation will be on the ballot again in 8 months. The following questions relate to this situation:

1. What would be the best thing for you, as a private practice dental hygienist, to do to help get the fluoride referendum passed?
   a. Continue educating your patients on the benefits of fluoride as you have been doing
   b. Start calling community leaders
   c. Make a financial contribution to the cause
   d. Wait and see what happens; you do not want to stir up the antifluoridationists
   e. Check with your local dental hygiene component to determine whether a unified plan of action has been developed and how you might help

2. The following political tactics will be beneficial in ensuring that the fluoridation referendum will pass except one:
   a. Public debate with the antifluoridationists
   b. Analysis of the referendum of 10 years ago
   c. Securing of an expert consultant to work with the professionals
   d. Endorsements by community leaders
   e. Distribution of literature in Spanish and English throughout the community

3. The best index to use to determine the decay rate in the elementary school–aged children would be:
   a. DMFT
   b. CPI
   c. OHI
   d. PDI
   e. GI

4. To make sure that your data will be reliable before you conduct the screening, you should:

   a. Contact the parents of the children

   b. Inform the children about oral hygiene

   c. Calibrate the examiners

   d. Plan how many children will be included

   e. Choose a stratified sample

5. If the fluoridation referendum fails to pass once again, which alternative plan would be the most effective?

   a. Sending letters to parents requesting them to take their children to the dentist for treatment and fluoride

   b. Giving oral hygiene lessons in the classrooms

   c. Initiating a school fluoride mouth rinse program

   d. Getting the children to participate in a sealant program

   e. Sending letters to parents about the benefits of fluoride

TESTLET NO. 2

You have recently been employed as a public health dental hygienist in a local health department. You have been asked to plan, implement, and evaluate a school-based educational and preventive program for selected elementary schools located in your school district. The program is to be based on the *Healthy People 2010* oral health objectives. Your plan includes classroom education and the use of a mobile dental van to provide cleanings, sealants, and fluorides. The following questions relate to the formation of this program.

1. All of the following are *Healthy People 2010* objectives that will be affected by your program except:

   a. Increasing the proportion of health departments that have an oral health component

   b. Increasing the proportion of children who receive sealants

   c. Increasing the proportion of children who are provided with topical fluoride

   d. Reducing the incidence of dental caries in children

   e. Reducing the incidence of periodontitis and gingivitis in children

2. Your planning includes collecting data using the DMFT Index. This tool of measurement will be helpful in assessing which of the following?

   a. The demand for services from your oral health program

   b. The amount of gingivitis and periodontitis in children's teeth

     c. The need for services from your oral health program

     d. The children's risk of contracting other health diseases

     e. The need for more dentists in your school district

3. In the evaluation phase of your program, you plan to measure the children's performance skills in the area of oral hygiene. Which method would be best to accomplish this?

     a. A written pretest and post-test

     b. A demonstration of the procedures by the children

     c. An oral survey of the children's attitudes on oral health

     d. A surprise index at the school after lunch

     e. A questionnaire for parents reporting on their children's brushing habits

4. On the dental van, you want to assess the needs of the children and make appropriate referrals for treatment. Which of the following methods would be best to relay to the parents the overall needs of their children after the screening?

     a. Sending the DMFT Index numbers home with the children

     b. Mailing literature on the importance of oral health to the parents

     c. Phoning the parents and report on the findings

     d. Sending a list of local dentists home with the children who need treatment

     e. Using the Basic Screening Survey (BSS) and sending the results home with a list of local community clinics

5. All of the these programs would be resources for payment in treating the children's teeth at the dentists' offices except:

     a. Medicare

     b. Medicaid

     c. State Children's Health Insurance Program (CHIP)

     d. Private insurance

     e. Head Start

TESTLET NO. 3

One of your private practice patients is a nursing home administrator. She requests your assistance in providing an oral health care program for the patients with Alzheimer's disease who reside at the Manor Care. The program is to include education, screening, and referral. The residents are from a lower socioeconomic group and have complex health histories. The social worker has consents for dental treatment, if needed, and a vehicle for transportation.

1. What would the first step be in planning this program?
    a. Arranging a time for an in-service for the nursing home staff
    b. Assessing survey attitudes of the residents to determine what is needed
    c. Arranging a meeting of the people to be involved to assess the needs and to determine goals and objectives for the program
    d. Determining which residents are receiving Medicare payments
    e. Planning an educational session for the residents

2. Which activity would be most beneficial to the goal of improving the residents' oral hygiene?
    a. Providing toothbrushes for the staff
    b. Purchasing electric toothbrushes for the residents
    c. Educating the staff on the importance of good oral hygiene self-care
    d. Educating the residents on oral diseases
    e. Showing the residents how to perform an oral cancer check

3. The screening indicates that there is a need for better oral hygiene and dental restorative work. All of the following are possibilities for dental care for the patients who are mobile except:
    a. Taking the elderly residents to a private practice dentist who accepts Medicare patients, since Medicare pays for dental treatment
    b. Checking with the nearby dental school for arranging to transport residents to their clinic for care on a reduced-fee or no-cost basis
    c. Taking the residents to a community clinic that bases its fees on a sliding scale
    d. Asking the dentist and hygienist in your community who use portable equipment to include Manor Care on their list of nursing homes to visit
    e. Discussing the problem with the local dental society to determine whether the members would be willing to participate in a community program to help the elderly receive dental care

4. The Gingival Index (GI) was performed on the residents with natural teeth. The following scores were recorded: 2.5, 2.7, 2.8, 3.0, 2.5, 2.4, and 2.9. Which score represents the mean GI score of the residents?
    a. 2.50
    b. 2.55
    c. 2.61

d. 2.63

e. 2.69

5. In analyzing the assessment data, the dental hygienist found the correlation between age and oral cancer to be +.80. This relationship could be described as:

a. Weak

b. Negative

c. Strong

d. Moderate

e. Not significant

TESTLET NO. 4

You reside in a small town and work in a community clinic. The regional public heath dental hygienist asks for your assistance in assessing, planning, and implementing oral health programs in your town. She is especially concerned about the elderly population and about developing a tobacco awareness program in the middle school.

1. You perform an assessment of the community's needs, including a description by age, gender, and socioeconomic status. This assessment is referred to as the:

a. Design of your plan

b. Community profile

c. List of priorities

d. Needs assessment

e. Problem definition

2. You decide to collect some baseline data to document the needs of the adults in the community and, possibly, to secure funds for program development. You want to measure healthy gingiva, presence or absence of bleeding, supragingival or subgingival calculus, and periodontal pockets. Which index would you use to screen the adults who visit your clinic?

a. OHI

b. DMFT

c. PDI

d. CPI

e. RCI

3. You intend to survey the middle school students to assess their perception of how susceptible they are to addiction and to cancer caused by

tobacco products. In your prevention program, you will present the benefits of not smoking or chewing and will discuss the results of their decisions. Which model of health promotion are you using?

a. Stages of Change Theory

b. Social Learning Theory

c. Community Organization Theory

d. Health Belief Model

e. Diffusion of Innovations Theory

4. Upon completion of your tobacco awareness program, you intend to present the results to other health care professionals at a health promotions meeting. Which strategy would you choose if you wish to reach a large number of people, have time for interaction, and do not intend to use AV equipment?

a. Poster presentation

b. Round table discussion

c. Oral paper

d. Table clinic

e. Written handout with your e-mail address on it

5. You bring your tobacco awareness program to the state public health dental hygienist. In attempting to follow the essential services of the public health core functions, the state dental hygienist wants to support and implement programs at all levels of prevention. At which level of prevention is your tobacco program?

a. Primary

b. Secondary

c. Tertiary

d. Planning

e. Implementing

Answers and rationales to the questions are presented next. Also see the chapters in which the information can be retrieved from within the text.

ANSWERS AND RATIONALES

The answers, rationales for each answer, and chapter cross-references are presented next.

Testlet No. 1

1. **e.** A unified plan of action is the best defense against a strong antifluoridation group. Anwers a., b., and c. are also possibilities of things you can do, but e. is best and foremost (see Chapter 5).

2. **a.** A public debate with antifluoridationists only provides them with an opportunity to reach more people with their scare tactics (see Chapter 5).

3. **a.** The DMFT Index is used to determine the decay rate in children (see Chapter 4).

4. **c.** Calibration of examiners is the best way to make sure that the data that you are collecting is reproducible or reliable (see Chapter 6).

5. **c.** A school fluoride mouth rinse program would be the next choice because it is inexpensive and would benefit all the children in reducing dental decay. Sealants are more expensive, and education does not guarantee a reduction in decay. These programs should be used in conjunction with fluoride (see Chapter 5).

Testlet No. 2

1. **e.** Reducing the incidence of periodontitis and gingivitis in children is not an objective of *Healthy People 2010*; all the other choices are objectives (see Chapter 4).

2. **c.** An assessment such as that conducted using the DMFT Index determines the *need* for oral health services. Answers b. and d. would not be appropriate because the DMFT Index is an assessment tool for determining decay. Although e. might be a conclusion, through critical thinking you can determine that this one single service probably is not the best solution (see Chapters 4 and 8).

3. **b.** Evaluation of performance is best conducted with an activity or demonstration by the person being evaluated (see Chapters 5 and 7).

4. **e.** The Basic Screening Survey is an easy tool to let parents know whether the child needs emergency care, whether treatment is necessary, or whether routine care is recommended. Local community clinics provide the best fee for service for low-income patients. It is

difficult to reach people by phone, and the follow-up list for referral is very important to the screening process (see Chapters 2 and 4).

5. **a.** Medicare is a program for elderly people, and it does not cover dental services. All of the other programs offer oral health treatment for children (see Chapter 5).

Testlet No. 3

1. **c.** Assessment of needs is always the first step in program planning (see Chapters 3 and 7).

2. **c.** The residents in nursing homes rely on the staff or caregivers to assist them with oral hygiene. Therefore, the staff must be educated on the importance of their own oral health first (see Chapters 2, 5, and 7).

3. **a.** All of these ideas would work except a., since Medicare does not offer dental benefits (see Chapter 5).

4. **e.** To find the mean, add the scores and divide by the total number of scores (see Chapter 6).

5. **c.** In comparing two variables, if the correlation is .7 or higher, the relationship is strong (see Chapter 6).

Testlet No. 4

1. **b.** "Community profile" is the term used to describe the community, including gender, age, and socioeconomic status (see Chapter 3).

2. **e.** The Community Periodontal Index (CPI) entails gathering data in all the areas described. It is a modification of the Community Periodontal Index of Treatment Needs (CPITN) and is more readily used. The other indices are too specific and not as inclusive. The PDI is not widely used anymore. (see Chapter 4).

3. **d.** The Health Belief Model is the only one listed that includes information on the people's perceptions or beliefs about oral health (see Chapter 7).

4. **a.** The poster presentation allows for the most interaction with the largest number of people. This is a popular presentation method at health promotion meetings. Audiovisual equipment is not used, and personal interaction is foremost (see Chapter 7).

5. **a.** Preventive services, such as a tobacco awareness program, are at the primary prevention level; they prevent the disease before it occurs. Secondary prevention reduces or eliminates disease in the early stages. Tertiary prevention limits disability from disease in later stages. Planning and implementing are phases of program development (see Chapters 1, 2, and 5).

Appendices

WEB SITES AND COMMUNITY RESOURCE LIST

Internet Web Addresses

American Dental Hygienists Association
(*http://www.adha.org*)

American Dental Assistants Association
(*http://members.aol.com/adaa1/index.html*)

Academy of General Dentistry
(*http://www.agd.org*)

American Dental Association
(*http://www.ada.org*)

American Public Health Association
(*http://www.apha.org*)

American Association of Public Health
Dentistry (*http://www.pitt.edu/~bjw/aaphd*)

Centers for Disease Control and
Prevention, Oral Health Division
(*http://www.cdc.gov/nccdphp/oh*)

Federation Dentaire Internationale (FDI)
World Dental Federation
(*http://www.fdi.org.uk*)

National Institute of Dental and
Craniofacial Research
(*http://www.nidcr.nih.gov*)

International and American Associations
for Dental Research (*http://www.iadr.com*)

World Health Organization
(*http://www.who.ch*)

American Medical Association
(*http://www.ama-assn.org*)

American Academy of Pediatric Dentistry
(*http://www.aapd.org*)

The American Academy of
Periodontology (*http://www.perio.org*)

American Association of Endodontists
(*http://www.aae.org*)

American Association of Orthodontists
(*http://www.aaortho.org*)

The American College of Prosthodontists
(*http://www.prosthodontics.org/acpros/index.htlm*)

Association of State and Territorial Dental
Directors (*http://www.astd.org*)

Synopsis of State Dental Public Health
Programs (*http://www.2.cdc.gov/nccdphp/doh/synopses/index.asp*)

U.S. Department of Health and Human
Services (*http://www.dhhs.gov*)

Occupational Safety and Health
Administration (OSHA)
(*http://www.osha.gov/oshinfo*)

National Oral Health Information
Clearinghouse
(*http://www.nohic.nidcr.nih.gov*)

Health Resources and Services
Administration (*http://www.hrsa.gov*)

Oral Health Initiative
(*http://www.hrsa.gov/oralhealth*)

National Maternal and Child Oral Health
Resource Center
(*http://www.ncemch.org/oralhealth*)

Children's Alliance (*http://www.
childrensalliance.org/teeth/coalition.htym*)

Block Drug Company
(*http://www.blockdrug.com*)

Colgate Company (*http://www.colgate.com*)

Procter & Gamble
(*http://www.dentalcare.com*)

Health Care Financing Administration
(HCFA) (*http://www.hcfa.gov*)

Oral Health America
(*http://www.oralhealthamerica.org*)

DENTAL HYGIENE COMPETENCIES

According to the "Competencies for Entry into the Profession of Dental Hygiene" American Association of Dental Schools Home of Delegates 1999 Annual Session, the dental hygienist must exhibit competencies in the five following domains:

1. The dental hygienist must possess, first, the **Core Competencies (C),** the ethics, values, skills, and knowledge integral to all aspects of the profession. These core competencies are foundational to all of the roles the dental hygienist.
2. Second, inasmuch as **Health Promotion (HP)** Disease Prevention is a key component of health care, changes within the health care environment require the dental hygienist to have a general knowledge of wellness, health determinants, and characteristics of various patient/client communities. The hygienist needs to emphasize both prevention of disease and effective health care delivery.
3. Third is the dental hygienist's complex role in the **Community (CM).** Dental hygienists must appreciate their role as health professionals at the local, state, and national levels. This role requires the graduate dental hygienist to assess, plan, and implement programs and activities to benefit the general population. In this role, the dental hygienist must be prepared to influence others to facilitate access to care and services.
4. Fourth is **Patient/Client Care (PC),** requiring competencies described here in ADPIE format. Because the dental hygienist's role in patient/client care is ever changing, yet central to the maintenance of health, dental hygiene graduates must use their skills to assess, diagnose, plan, implement, and evaluate treatment.
5. Fifth, like other health professionals, dental hygienists must be aware of a variety of opportunities for **Professional Growth and Development (PGD).** Some opportunities may increase clients' access to dental hygiene; others may offer ways to influence the profession and the changing health care environment. A dental hygienist must possess transferable skills (e.g., in communication, problem solving, and critical thinking) to take advantage of these opportunities.

Core Competencies

C.1 Apply a professional code of ethics in all endeavors.

C.2 Adhere to state and federal laws, recommendations, and regulations in the provision of dental hygiene care.

C.3 Provide dental hygiene care to promote patient/client health and wellness using critical thinking and problem solving in the provision of evidenced-based practice.

C.4 Assume responsibility for dental hygiene actions and care based on accepted scientific theories and research as well as the accepted standard of care.

C.5 Continuously perform self-assessment for lifelong learning and professional growth.

C.6 Advance the profession through service activities and affiliations with professional organizations.

C.7 Provide quality assurance mechanisms for health services.

C.8 Communicate effectively with individuals and groups from diverse populations both verbally and in writing.

C.9 Provide accurate, consistent, and complete documentation for assessment, diagnosis, planning, implementation, and evaluation of dental hygiene services.

C.10 Provide care to all clients using an individualized approach that is humane, empathetic, and caring.

Health Promotion and Disease Prevention

HP.1 Promote the values of oral and general health and wellness to the public and organizations within and outside the profession.

HP.2 Respect the goals, values, beliefs, and preferences of the patient or client while promoting optimal oral and general health.

HP.3 Refer patients or clients who may have a physiologic, psychological, or social problem for comprehensive patient and client evaluation.

HP.4 Identify individual and population risk factors, and develop strategies that promote health-related quality of life.

HP.5 Evaluate factors that can be used to promote patient or client adherence to disease prevention or health maintenance strategies.

HP.6 Evaluate and utilize methods to ensure the health and safety of the patient or client and the dental hygienist in the delivery of dental hygiene.

Community Involvement

CM.1 Assess the oral health needs of the community and the quality and availability of resources and services.

CM.2 Provide screening, referral, and educational services that allow clients to access the resources of the health care system.

CM.3 Provide community oral health services in a variety of settings.

CM.4 Facilitate client access to oral health services by influencing individuals and organizations for the provision of oral health care.

CM.5 Evaluate reimbursement mechanisms and their impact on the patient or client's access to oral health care.

CM.6 Evaluate the outcomes of community-based programs, and plan for future activities.

Patient and Client Care

Assessment

PC.1 Systematically collect, analyze, and record data on the general, oral, and psychosocial health status of a variety of patients or clients using methods consistent with medicolegal principles.

   This competency includes the following steps:

a. Select, obtain, and interpret diagnostic information, recognizing its advantages and limitations.

b. Recognize predisposing and etiologic risk factors that require intervention to prevent disease.

c. Obtain, review, and update a complete medical, family, social, and dental history.
d. Recognize health conditions and medications that affect overall patient or client care.
e. Identify patients or clients at risk for a medical emergency, and manage the patient or client care in a manner that prevents an emergency.
 f. Perform a comprehensive examination using clinical, radiographic, periodontal, dental charting, and other data collection procedures to assess the patient's or clients needs.

Diagnosis
PC.2 Use critical decision-making skills to reach conclusions about the patient's or client's dental hygiene needs based on all available assessment data.
 This competency includes the following steps:
a. Use assessment findings, etiologic factors, and clinical data in determining a dental hygiene diagnosis.
b. Identify patient or client needs and significant findings that affect the delivery of dental hygiene services.
c. Obtain consultations as indicated.

Planning
PC.3 Collaborate with the patient or client, or other health professionals to formulate a comprehensive dental hygiene care plan that is patient-centered or client-centered and based on current scientific evidence.
 This competency includes the following steps:
a. Prioritize the care plan based on the health status and the actual and potential problems of the individual to facilitate optimal oral health.
b. Establish a planned sequence of care (educational, clinical, and evaluation) based on the dental hygiene diagnosis; identified oral conditions; potential problems; etiologic and risk factors; and available treatment modalities.
c. Establish a collaborative relationship with the patient or client in the planned care to include etiology, prognosis, and treatment alternatives.
d. Make referrals to other health care professionals.
e. Obtain the patient's or client's informed consent based on a thorough case presentation.

Implementation
PC.4 Provide specialized treatment that includes preventive and therapeutic services designed to achieve and maintain oral health. Assist in achieving oral health goals formulated in collaboration with the patient/client.
 This competency includes the following steps:
a. Perform dental hygiene interventions to eliminate or control local etiologic factors to prevent and control caries, periodontal disease, and other oral conditions.
b. Control pain and anxiety during treatment through the use of accepted clinical and behavioral techniques.
c. Provide life support measures to manage medical emergencies in the patient or client care environment.

Evaluation
PC.5 Evaluate the effectiveness of the implemented clinical, preventive, and educational services, and modify as needed.

This competency includes the following steps:

a. Determine the outcomes of dental hygiene interventions using indices, instruments, examination techniques, and the patient or client self-report.
b. Evaluate the patient's or client's satisfaction with the oral health care received and the oral health status achieved.
c. Provide subsequent treatment or referrals based on evaluation findings.
d. Develop and maintain a health maintenance program.

Professional Growth and Development

PGD.1　Identify alternative career options within health care, industry, education, and research, and evaluate the feasibility of pursuing dental hygiene opportunities.

PGD.2　Develop management and marketing strategies to be used in nontraditional health care settings.

PGD.3　Access professional and social networks and resources to assist entrepreneurial initiatives.

The American Association of Dental Schools (now called the American Dental Education Association) drafted these competency statements. Representation was provided from both baccalaureate and associate degree dental hygiene programs. It also included representation from dental hygiene, clinical, social, and basic sciences and the American Dental Hygienists Association. A separate committee, the Dental Hygiene Education Competency Draft Review Committee, further reviewed and provided feedback on the document. The competency statements were presented for public comment at the 1998 AADS Annual Session, the 1998 Dental Hygiene Directors conference, and the Section on Dental Hygiene Education home page on the World Wide Web.

Bibliography

American Association of Dental Schools (ADDS): Competencies for Entry into Profession of Dental Hygiene: Washington, DC, AADS Section on Dental Hygiene Education; approved March 1999.

POTENTIAL COMMUNITY PARTNERS

Health Groups, Organizations, and Associations

- Dental Professional Associations
- American Academy of Pediatrics (AAP)
- American Medical Association (AMA)
- American Nurses Association (ANA)
- State and local health professional societies
- Emergency department technicians
- Nurse Midwives
- Private pediatric practices

- Health maintenance organizations (HMOs), Health Insurance Companies
- Hospitals, health systems, nursing homes, senior centers
- Maternity care
- Community health centers
- Schools of public health
- Health Associations (American Cancer Society, United Cerebral Palsy)

Government Agencies and Programs

- Health departments
- Americorps
- Human service agencies, protective service agencies
- Department of Agriculture, Extension Service
- Department of Education

- Department of Motor Vehicles
- State, local, and tribal governments
- Nutrition and Women, Infants, and Children (WIC)
- Elected officials
- Community planning

Community Organizations

- Community foundations
- Community information and resource centers
- Junior League
- Rotary International
- Red Cross
- Kiwanis
- Lions

- Elks
- Healthy Mothers/Healthy Babies Coalitions
- Religious organizations
- Salvation Army
- Drug and Alcohol Resistance Education Programs (DARE)
- Alcoholics Anonymous (AA)

- United Way
- YMCA, YWCA
- Big Brothers/Big Sisters
- March of Dimes

- Homeless organizations
- Minority organizations
- Service organizations for elderly, disabled, veterans, women, and youth

Education-Related Organizations and Groups

- American Federation of Teachers (AFT)
- National Education Association (NEA)
- Adult and continuing education programs
- School districts and boards
- Home school programs
- Fraternities and sororities
- Alumni organizations
- Head Start programs and day care centers

- Recreation facilities and programs
- Literacy programs
- Retired teachers
- Colleges and universities
- Employment and vocational training
- Parenting education
- Parent-Teacher Associations

Advocacy Organizations

- Council of La Raza
- Children's Defense Fund
- National Association for the Advancement of Colored People (NAACP)
- Urban League
- American Association of Retired Persons (AARP)
- Special Olympics
- Association for Retarded Citizens (ARC)

- League of Women Voters
- Community coalitions, collaborations, and initiatives
- Coalition for Asian-American Children and Families
- National Resource Center on Native American Aging

Business Organizations and Retail Outlets

- Airlines
- Banks
- Beauty and barber shops
- Chambers of commerce
- Computer companies and stores
- Grocery stores
- Delicatessens, specialty and ethnic food stores

- Health clubs
- Insurance companies
- Shopping malls
- Maternity stores
- Movie theaters

Adapted from Seven Days of Immunizations: National Infant Immunization Week, U.S. Department of Health and Human Services, Public Health Service. Atlanta, Centers for Disease Control and Prevention, 1995.

RESOURCES FOR COMMUNITY HEALTH ASSESSMENT

Examples of Information for a Community Profile

Physical and Spatial Characteristics

Geopolitical boundaries, community-designated boundaries, geographic size, community location description, population size, population density, community type, general physical environment, geographical isolation, physical conditions of neighborhoods, community assets, people-made environment, layout of the community, residential neighborhoods, business districts, buildings, greenspace, parks, transportation routes, roads, traffic, congestion, environmental conditions, air quality, water supply, water quality, community infrastructure, education resources and facilities, location and characteristics of local institutions, landmarks, art, media, playgrounds, recreation facilities and resources, libraries, public commons and informal gathering places, number of places of worship, religious denominations, local economy and types of industry, signs of development or decay in community areas, patterns of day-to-day activities and everyday human interactions

Community Inventory

History of community, community traditions, dominant values, significant beliefs, events that have occurred in the community with a short-term or long-term effect on the health of the community, political system, local government structure, political structure, dominant political affiliation, number of registered voters, power structure, formal and informal community leadership, formal community support systems, informal helping networks/mutual support and trusted community members, gatekeepers, opinion leaders, community historians, communication channels, inventories of citizen's associations and community organizations, inventory of capacities of individual community members and groups of individuals

Sociodemographic Characteristics

Community Demographic Data

Population distribution by age, gender, race and ethnicity composition, social class, economic status, education levels, occupations, religions, marital status; gender ratios, socioeconomic data, employment status, neighborhood living conditions, value of housing, household living conditions, household crowding, indices of deprivation, levels of education, religion, nationality, and cultural characteristics, generational information, in-migration and out-migration, immigration status, trends of change in size and composition

Social Demographic Data

Social attributes, social structure, community stability, social cohesiveness, civic engagement and pride, social networks, family and household characteristics, family values, family living patterns, community norms, customs, and lifestyles, health-enhancing behaviors, values, attitudes, beliefs, opinions, social forces, cultural forces, religious beliefs, enrollment in government programs (including Temporary Assistance for Needy Families [TANF]), public assistance, food stamps, Supplemental Food Program for Women, Infants, and Children (WIC), Head Start, child care support, Medicaid, Children's Health Insurance Program (S-CHIP), vulnerable populations groups in community, quality of life, crime and security

Vital Events

Natality (births), fertility rates, life expectancy, mortality (deaths), marriages, divorces, population mobility

APPENDIX D-2

Examples of Government Resources for Health Data

- Bureau of the Census, Department of Commerce
- Bureau of Labor Statistics, Department of Labor, state employment security office
- National Vital Statistics System (NVSS), state and local vital records (natality [birth], mortality [death], marriage, and divorce certificates)
- National Notifiable Diseases Surveillance System, national, state, and local communicable disease reports and records
- Behavioral Risk Factor Surveillance Survey conducted by Behavioral Risk Factor Surveillance System (BRFSS) at CDC, states (state-based telephone survey), and localities
- Youth Risk Behavior Survey (YRBS) conducted by Youth Risk Behavior Surveillance System (YRBSS), (CDC), school-based survey of high school students
- Pregnancy Risk Assessment Monitoring System (PRAMS), CDC, population-based surveillance system states use to monitor selected maternal attitudes, behaviors, and experiences
- State Cancer Registries (CDC) and Cancer Registry with the Surveillance, Epidemiology and End Results Program (SEER), National Cancer Institute
- Water Fluoridation Reporting System (WFRS) Census, CDC
- National Health Interview Survey (NHIS)
- National Health and Nutrition Examination Survey (NHANES)
- Medical Expenditure Panel Survey (MEPS)

- School Health Policies and Programs Study (SHPPS), CDC
- National Nursing Home Survey
- National Profile of Local Health Departments (NPLHD)
- Medicare Statistical System
- Medicaid Data System
- U.S. Environmental Protection Agency, state environmental quality agency, local environment agency

<u>APPENDIX D–3</u>

Examples of Information for a Community Health Assessment

Community Health Measures	Examples
Health Status (measurements of natality [births], morbidity [illness], and mortality [deaths])	*Birth statistics:* Age, parity of mother, duration of pregnancy, types of births (single, twin), complications of pregnancy, complications of birth, birth defects, birth weight (e.g., low), premature births, births to adolescent, older, or unmarried females *Morbidity statistics:* Incidence and prevalence of diseases, conditions, disabilities, or injuries (distribution, intensity, and duration), such as unintentional and intentional injuries, homicide, suicide, cancer, heart disease, diabetes, stroke, infectious diseases (communicable) HIV/AIDS, tuberculosis, STDs, mental illness, alcohol and drug abuse problems, occupational diseases, disability and decreased independence, developmental disabilities (e.g., cleft lip and/or palate, craniofacial anomalies), oral diseases or conditions (e.g., dental caries, periodontal diseases, oral injuries) *Mortality statistics:* Distribution of death rates by age, race/ethnicity, sex, cause, geographic location, leading causes of deaths such as cancer (breast, colon, lung, oral), heart disease, stroke, homicide, motor vehicle injuries, suicide, unintentional injury, infant, neonatal, and postneonatal mortality
Health risks and protective factors (identification of patterns of behavioral and nonbehavioral factors)	Self-rated (self-reported) general and oral health status, recent poor health, days of work lost, days of school lost (e.g., due to dental problems or care), average number of unhealthy days in past month, satisfaction with quality of life and with public health, health care, and social service system

(continues)

Community Health *continued*

Measures	Examples
	Occupational risks and work disability

Stress indicators and resources (drunk driving, robberies, assaults), access to drugs, recent drug use, alcoholic beverage outlets, gang problems, family violence (child abuse and neglect, spouse and elder abuse), major depression, self-esteem, alienation, discrimination, feelings of hope and despair, feelings of anger, social and family support, social and family resources (adaptation and cohesion), life events, stress (personal, family, job stress)

Levels of health knowledge, beliefs, attitudes, behaviors, practices, and skills about self-care (toothbrushing with fluoride toothpaste and flossing) and health interventions, lifestyle diet (low in sugar), physical activity, health-related substance use (tobacco and alcohol), safety practices (seat belts, mouth guards), knowledge about location and availability as well as appropriate use of local health resources, services, programs, family health care expenditures

Use of child and adult preventive health services: dental sealants, fluoride treatments, prenatal care in first trimester, immunizations for children and adults, Pap smear, mammogram, sigmoidoscopy for colon cancer screening

Access to public health, health care and social service system (scope, adequacy, accessibility, and availability of services in a coordinated, integrated system)

Access to community preventive services (community water fluoridation) and public health services: Scope and adequacy of local health department covering essential public health services (including infrastructure and capacity measures, local voluntary health programs, operational health promotion and education programs in work sites, schools, and community) by health providers, numbers, types, locations, adequacy

Access to facilities for personal health care: Assessment of numbers, types, location, adequacy of hospitals, emergency facilities, outpatient primary care, oral health, hearing, vision care, speech, physical, and occupational therapy, urgent care, mental health, alcohol and drug treatment programs, nursing homes, community health centers

Access to health professionals: Adequacy and numbers of trained public health professionals and personal health service professionals with expertise and competence, levels of knowledge,

> attitudes, and behaviors, practices, and skills of public health professionals and personal health service professionals
>
> **_Access to health insurance and usual sources of health care:_** Comprehensive benefits with dental insurance and per capita spending (Medicare, Medicaid, state Children's Health Insurance Program [CHIP], private insurance, Supplementary Security Income)
>
> Scope and adequacy of local social service programs in addressing basic human family and community needs

AIDS, acquired immunodeficiency disease; HIV, human immunodeficiency virus; STD, sexually transmitted disease

APPENDIX D–4

Examples of Primary Data Collection Tasks

Planning

- Determine scope and objectives
- Prepare protocols describing assessment plan
- Select data collection methods
- Establish criteria
- Determine sampling methods and processes
- Obtain approval of authorities
- Plan for personnel and physical arrangements
- Plan for data analysis phase (recording, managing, and analyzing data)
- Plan for data reporting phase
- Prepare budget
- Develop timetable of main activities and responsible staff
- Plan for referral process (for clinical findings detected in health survey)
- Plan and develop consent form
- Translate consent form
- Gain approval of consent form from Institutional Review Board
- Plan and develop data collection instruments
- Plan and develop data collection and entry process (manual collection or direct data entry into personal computer)
- Translate data collection instruments
- Gain approval of data collection instruments from Institutional Review Board
- Pilot test consent form and data collection instruments
- Revise consent form and data collection instruments
- Obtain approval of revised consent form and data collection instruments from Institutional Review Board
- Draw sample
- Plan fieldwork and scheduling
- Purchase and organize supplies
- Initiate contact with data collection sites (work through established community networks or organizational structures)
- Organize logistics for data collection, including travel and site requirements

- Develop data collection protocols
- Plan data entry processes
- Plan quality assurance processes for data collection
- Plan and develop training materials for field team

- Train field team
- Calibrate field team
- Implement pilot test of assessment

Implementing

- Contact and recruit participants
- Gain consent of participants
- Record data
- Manage data

- Analyze data
- Maintain quality assurance processes
- Summarize findings
- Report findings

Glossary

Abstract A summary, confined to approximately 200 words, that concisely defines a study's purpose, methods, materials, and results; a brief description of the research, found at the beginning of a manuscript, designed to provide an overview of the study

Access Assurance that conditions are in place for people to obtain the care they need and want

Administrator or **Manager** A supervisory role in which the dental hygienist directs and oversees oral health programs

Agent Factors Biological or mechanical means of causing disease, illness, injury, or disability, including microbial, parasitic, viral, and bacterial pathogens or vectors; physical or mechanical irritants; chemicals; drugs; trauma; automobiles; and radiation

Alternative Practice A setting outside the private office in which the dental hygienist provides public health services

ANOVA (Analysis of Variance) A commonly used test for parametrics; allows comparison among more than two means from different samples and compares interactions among the variability in multiple sample groups to the variability within groups

Assessment A core public health function that includes the regular and systematic collection, assemblage, and analysis of data and communication regarding the oral health of the community

ASTDD (Association of State and Territorial Dental Directors) Basic Screening Survey A survey used to assess need and referral for dental care; categories include (1) no dental care needed other than routine care, (2) early dental care recommended, and (3) urgent or emergency care recommended

Assurance A core public health function in which agencies educate, support, and evaluate programs to ensure that the community's oral health needs are addressed

BRFSS (Behavioral Risk Factor Surveillance Survey) A state-specific survey developed by the Centers for Disease Control and Prevention; structured questions are asked over the telephone to assess behaviors that influence health status; an oral health module assesses utilization of dental services

Calibration   Agreement of examiners who are involved in data collection with a set standard of performance

Change Agent/Consumer Advocate   A role in which the dental hygienist must have the knowledge and skills to work to promote change and advance people's health through legislation, public policy, research, and science

Chi-Square Test   The most commonly used nonparametric test; is used to analyze questionnaire data and to determine whether a relationship exists between two variables

Community   The public or group of people with common interests who live in a specific locality

Community Oral Health Assessment   A multifaceted process of identifying factors that affect the oral health of a selected population in order to determine resources and interventions for oral health improvement

Community Organization Theory   The idea of involving and activating members of a community or subgroup to identify a common problem or goal, to mobilize resources, to implement strategies, and to evaluate their efforts

Community Profile   A comprehensive description of the community, including items such as population size, geographic boundaries, community type, and physical conditions

Community Water Fluoridation   The addition of a controlled amount of fluoride to the public water supply with the intent of preventing dental caries in the population

Consult/Resource Person   A role in which the dental hygienist acts as a liaison between the community and the dental profession to determine the appropriate programs and activities that will serve the needs of the community

Continuous Data   A type of collected information described as measurements made from a particular value, such as from temperature, scores on tests, or time; can be any value along a continuum

Control Group   The group of subjects in a study who do not receive the experimental treatment or intervention

Convenience Sample   A group of individuals who are most readily available to be subjects in a study

Correlation   A statistical method of determining whether a variation in one variable may be related to a variation in another variable

CPI (Community Periodontal Index) An assessment of periodontal status of a population by grades of periodontal disease; measures gingival bleeding, calculus, and periodontal pockets

Cultural Competence Considerations that have an impact on the profession's responsibility to reduce the burden of disease for people of various cultures and backgrounds

Current Status State of affairs or position at the present time

Data Pieces of information collected from measurements and counts obtained during the course of a research study

Data Collection The process of gathering the information that can be used by the community to make decisions and set priorities

Demand Health care services desired by the individual or community

Dental Public Health The science and art of preventing and controlling dental disease and promoting dental health through organized community efforts

DHHS (Department of Health and Human Services) A department of the federal government presiding over agencies that conduct oral health activities

Dependent Variable The variable thought to depend on or to be caused by the independent variable; the outcome variable of interest

Descriptive Statistics Used to describe and summarize data; determine information only about the sample being studied

Determinants of Health Factors that interact to create circumstances and produce specific health conditions; can be classified as physical (environmental), biologic, behavioral, social, cultural, and spiritual

Diffusion of Innovations Theory A concept that assesses how new ideas, products, or services spread within a society or to other groups or how innovations are adopted

Discrete Data Collected information that is counted only in whole numbers

Disparities Uneven distribution of the burden of oral diseases throughout the population, especially in the poor, the elderly, and the disabled

DMFT, DMFS (Decayed, Missing, and Filled Teeth/Surfaces) Index A survey used to count caries in the permanent dentition; **dft** and **dfs** are used to count caries in the primary dentition

Environmental Factors Physical, sociocultural, sociopolitical, and economic components that interact with host and agent

Epidemiology   The study of the distribution and determinants of health-related states and events in specified populations and the application of this study to the control of health problems

Essential Public Health Services for Oral Health   Guidelines describing the roles of state oral health programs; used in the development and evaluation of public health activities at the state level

Ethics/Professional Ethics   The general science of right and wrong conduct; the code by which the profession regulates actions and sets standards for its members

Evaluation   The method of measuring results of a program against objectives developed during the early planning stages

Experimental Group   The sample group of subjects in a study who receive the experimental treatment or intervention

Focus Group   Five to 10 members of the intended target audience who undergo group interviews lasting about 30 to 60 minutes; a moderator with structured questions guides the discussion

Follow-up/Referral   An essential component of assessment and screening; without further observation and referral for care, screening is ineffective

Framing Health Messages   A concept that relates to the cues (e.g., sounds, symbols, words, pictures) that signal how and what to think about an issue

General Supervision   Supervision of the dental hygienist in which the dentist does not have to be on the premises but the patient must be one of record or seen by the dentist previously

Goal   A broad-based statement of changes to take place from which specific objectives are developed

Health   Complete physical and social well-being, not merely the absence of disease

Health Belief Model   An assessment of perceptions of how susceptible one is to a health problem and whether one believes that recommended preventive behaviors will result in less susceptibility

Health Education   The process in which the client is encouraged to become responsible for personal oral health and is informed of scientifically based methods for preventing dental disease

Health Educator/Wellness Promoter   A role in which the dental hygienist works to prevent disease and to promote oral health through the presentation of scientific information

Health Promotion A broad concept referring to the process of enabling people and communities to increase their control over the determinants of health and, therefore, to improve their own health

Health Security The rights and conditions that enable individuals to attain and enjoy their full potential for a healthy life

Healthy People 2010 A document that contains national health objectives for prevention of disease and promotion of health

Host Factors Factors that affect a host's (a person's, an animal's, or a plant's) susceptibility and resistance to disease

Hypothesis A statement that reflects the research question, stated in positive terms, and represents the researcher's prediction or opinion

Implementation The process of putting a plan into action; monitoring a plan's activities, personnel, equipment, resources, and supplies

Independent Variable The experimental treatment or intervention that is imposed on the experimental group

Index A graduated numeric scale with upper and lower limits; scores correspond to a specific criterion for individuals or populations

Inferential Statistics Used to draw a generalization between the sample studied and the actual population

Interrater Reliability Agreement of findings by two or more examiners

Interval Scale A scale of measurement that determines quantities; characterized by having order and equal distance between points on the scale

Intrarater Reliability Consistency of findings by one examiner with those previously recorded by the same examiner

Judgmental Sample A sample, provided through personal judgment, of subjects who are most representative of the population

Learning Styles The ways in which people collect and retain knowledge

Legislative/Policy Changes New or revised laws on health care that the dental hygienist as Consumer Advocate/Change Agent helps to create and implement

Mandala of Health Hancock's model of health of the human ecosystem

Mean Average of the group; a sum of all the values divided by the number of items

Median The exact middle score or value in a distribution of scores; when the total number of scores is even, the sum of the two middle scores, divided by 2, provides the median

Mode   The score or value that occurs most frequently in a distribution of scores

Need   Those services deemed by the health professional to be necessary after use of a variety of assessment and diagnostic tools and, perhaps, past experience

Network   A system in which information about a common population is shared with other health professionals

NHANES (National Health and Nutrition Examination Survey)   A national survey conducted in 1996 in which many aspects of oral health were measured

NHIS (National Health Interview Survey)   A survey that asks questions about a person's health, including edentulous status

Nominal Scale   A scale of measurement in which characteristics or numbers are assigned into categories by name only

Nonparametric Test   A statistical test used when assumptions about a normal distribution in the population cannot be met or when the level of measurement is nominal or ordinal

Normal Distribution   An assumption that approximately 68% of the population falls within 1 standard deviation (SD) of the mean, approximately 95% falls within 2 SDs of the mean, and 99% lies within 3 SDs of the mean

Null Hypothesis   An assumption that there is no statistically significant difference between the groups being studied

Objective   The desired end result of program activities, described in a measurable way; more specific than a goal

Oral Health Coalition   A cooperative effort on the part of many individuals and organizations to build systems and to develop programs that improve community oral health

Oral Health Education   A learning experience directed at assisting people in preventing oral disease

Oral Paper   A method of presentation of a topic

Ordinal Scale   A scale of measurement that orders data into categories in rank order; the space between these categories is undefined

Organizational Change: Stage Theory   A statement of how organizations pass through a series of stages as they initiate change; organizational structures and processes influence workers' behavior and motivation for change

Parameter   A term relating to numeric characteristics of the population

Parametrics A technique used when data include interval or ratio scales of measurement; best used when the sample is large and randomized and the population from which the sample is taken is normally distributed

Pilot Study (Trial Run) A preliminary study performed in preparation for a major study

Planning An organized response to reduce or eliminate one or more problems

Planning Cycle A model commonly used in public health practice that provides a basic flow chart of steps in process to assess, plan, implement, and evaluate

Pluralistic Systems Numerous, distinct health care delivery systems that coexist simultaneously

Policy Development A core public health function in which laws are planned and developed to support community oral health issues

Population The entire group, or whole unit of individuals, having similar characteristics to which the results of an investigation can be generalized

Poster A method of presentation of a topic

Power Analysis A determination of how many subjects are needed to provide significance; calculated using a specific statistical formula based on what an examiner hopes to observe in a specific number of subjects

Primary Prevention Services that are used to prevent a disease before it occurs; this level includes health education, avoidance of disease, and health protection

Professional Ethics The code by which the profession regulates actions and sets standards for its members

Public Health The science and art of preventing disease, prolonging life, and promoting physical health and efficiency through organized community effort

***P* Value** A declaration of how likely it is that a study could have come to a false conclusion; the probability that the obtained results are due to chance alone

Qualitative Data Information that reflects the quality or nature of things that cannot be numerically measured or analyzed

Qualitative Evaluation A determination of why and, how (e.g., why did people participate in the activity, and how do they intend to change their parenting behaviors?)

Quality of Life Characteristics of living that are affected by a person's health status; oral disease restricts activities at school, work, and home and often diminishes one's quality of life

Quantitative Data Information that is objective and measurable; can be expressed in a quantity or amount (such as the number of children with dental sealants or the rate of dental caries in young children)

Quantitative Evaluation A determination of how many (e.g., how many people increased their knowledge of the causes of early childhood caries?)

Random Sample A sample in which each member of a population has an equal chance of being included, thus preventing the possibility of selection bias by the researcher

Range A measurement of the difference between the highest and lowest values in a distribution of scores

Ratio Scale A scale of measurement that not only has all the qualities of nominal, ordinal, and interval but also has an absolute zero, such as age, height, and weight

Refereed Journal A journal in which articles have been reviewed by an editorial board of peers

Reliability Consistency and stability of the data collected in a study

Researcher A role in which the dental hygienist uses scientific methods to acquire knowledge on topics relevant to serving the needs of the public's oral health

Round Table Discussion Method of presentation of a topic in which the participants sit in a circular pattern and discuss issues relevant to the topic

Sample A portion or subset of the entire population

Sealant A plastic resin material applied to the occlusal surfaces of molars and premolars; an effective primary preventive strategy

Service-Learning Programs Often referred to as *extramural rotations;* programs using structured learning experiences designed by faculty and community member teams with students providing direct services to groups with identified needs

Service Provider/Clinician A role in which the dental hygienist assesses oral health needs and provides treatment

Shortage Areas Localities where the dentist-to-population ratio shows an unmet need for oral health

Social Learning Theory The idea that people learn through their own experiences by observing the actions of others and the results of those actions

Social Marketing Use of effective advertising tools from commercial marketing to influence a valued health behavioral change

Social Responsibility A broad term encompassing professionalism, personal and professional ethics, and the role of a profession in the context of the greater society

Stages of Change Theory The idea that change is a process or cycle that occurs over time rather than as a single event

Standard Deviation The positive square root of the variance

Statistics Numeric characteristics of samples

Status State or condition

Stratified Sample Random selection of subjects from two or more subdivisions of the population

Systematic Approach to Health Improvement Framework describing the interrelated determinants of health, including the goals and objectives necessary to improve health

Systematic Sample Selection of subjects by including every nth person in a list

Table Clinic Method of presentation of a topic

Tailoring Messages A concept in which specific cues are used to make messages meaningful for a specific individual

Target Population The people from whom the information is being collected and to whom the researcher would like to generalize the findings of a study

Technical Assistance The use of the professional skills and knowledge base to provide guidance to nondental community members interested in developing preventive programs

Theory A set of interrelated concepts, definitions, and propositions that present a systematic view of events or situations by specifying relations among variables in order to explain and predict the events or situations

Trend Inclination or direction on a particular course over a period of time

t-Test A test used to analyze the difference between two means

Type I (Alpha) Error On the basis of statistical results, the researcher rejects the null hypothesis when it is true

Type II (Beta) Error On the basis of statistical results, the researcher accepts the null hypothesis when it is actually false

Validity The degree to which an instrument measures what it is intended to measure

Variable A characteristic or concept that varies, or differs, within the population under study

Variance A method of measuring the way in which individual variables are located around the mean; a common technique of measuring interval and ratio variables

Index

Note: Page numbers followed by the letter f refer to figures; those followed by the letter b refer to boxes, and those followed by the letter t refer to tables.